D0500224

# Menopause
# and Madness

# Menopause and Madness

## The Truth About Estrogen and the Mind

Marcia Lawrence

**Andrews McMeel**
**Publishing**

Kansas City

*Menopause and Madness* copyright © 1998 by Marcia Lawrence.
All rights reserved. Printed in the United States of America.
No part of this book may be used or reproduced in any manner
whatsoever except in the case of reprints in the context of reviews.
For information, write Andrews McMeel Publishing, an
Andrews McMeel Universal company,
4520 Main Street, Kansas City, Missouri 64111.

www.andrewsmcmeel.com

98 99 00 01 RDH 10 9 8 7 6 5 4 3 2 1

Library of Congress Cataloging-in-Publication Data

Lawrence, Marcia
Menopause and madness : the truth about estrogen
and the mind / Marcia Lawrence
p.    cm.
Includes bibliographical references.
ISBN 0-8362-3592-4
1. Menopause—Psychological aspects. 2. Menopause—Hormone therapy.
3. Estrogen—Therapeutic use. I. Title.
RG186.L39  1998
618.1'75'0019—dc21      97-36399
CIP

Attention: Schools and Businesses

Andrews McMeel books are available at quantity discounts
with bulk purchase for educational, business, or sales promotional use.
For information, please write to: Special Sales Department,
Andrews McMeel Publishing, 4520 Main Street,
Kansas City, Missouri 64111.

*For*
*Ralph N. Wharton, M.D.*

*The force that through the green fuse drives the flower*
—Dylan Thomas

# Contents

# Contents

# Preface

# My Story . . . and Yours

On August 28, 1985, I became engulfed in a maelstrom of insanity that spanned seventeen days and nearly destroyed me. I was helpless against biological forces that overpowered my mind and rendered me defenseless. I became a menopause casualty.

For a couple of years I had suffered from a number of vague physical symptoms. They were unfamiliar to me, and I wasn't able to interpret them. Sometimes I would feel a crawling sensation up and down my legs, as though there were something moving under my skin. I also experienced occasional tingling and numbness in my fingers. I didn't know what it was; I just wasn't feeling quite right. The doctors whom I saw were unable to find any obvious problem. Although the physical sensations were annoying, I wasn't depressed, nor did I exhibit any of the usual symptoms associated with depression. I had no difficulty concentrating. There were no feelings of hopelessness or lassitude. To the contrary, my energy level was high. The early summer of 1985 was busy as always, filled with outdoor concerts, summer theater, entertaining friends and family, and teaching part-time. I was forty-nine and in my prime. The notion that, in a matter of months, my life would spin out of control was unthinkable.

Yet, late on that August afternoon, in one explosive moment, my brain seemed to short-circuit. It was as if all the connecting neuro-transmitters suddenly malfunctioned, plunging me into a delusional world. For what seemed an eternity—but miraculously lasted only two and a half weeks—I became isolated inside my head and accepted unquestioningly the power of otherworldly voices which guided and ruled my life. I existed in an altered reality. Only after days of psychosis that led me to the brink of death did I learn the truth. I had gone mad from estrogen deprivation.

Even as I write these words, I know I am entering highly controversial territory. There has been an organized campaign to prevent the words *estrogen* and *madness* from ever appearing in the same sentence. This campaign is waged by women's organizations, whose views I normally share, out of fear that this discussion will breathe new life into the archaic belief that all women are driven crazy by their hormones. It also is waged by cancer experts, like Dr. Susan Love, who have their own agendas when it comes to recommending estrogen treatment. And it is waged by psychiatrists and gynecologists, each side fearing a loss of territory to the other.

So while much of the mainstream medical establishment continues to deny the connection between psychiatric illness and the biochemical changes that occur in menopause, the potential for tragedy is great. Out of approximately seventy million menopausal women, 15 percent—10.5 million women—are rendered mentally dysfunctional. In such a condition, suicide becomes a real risk. There are women who are enduring frightening depressive episodes, committing bizarre and often horribly violent acts because of their bodies' sensitivity to changes in their estrogen levels.

I am writing this book to let women know there is another

side—a side I can speak about credibly, both from my own experience and from my extensive research. The truth that so many
people fear is this: Certain women have a special sensitivity to declining levels of estrogen that triggers a systemic malfunction. Scientists have been slow to identify the phenomenon, and they are
only now beginning to understand the enormous influence of estrogen.

Estrogen is not an isolated hormone related solely to fertility. It
is ubiquitous, secreted directly into the bloodstream and tissues of
the body. Its effect on blood chemistry, bones, and the vascular system is far-reaching. Estrogen is carried through a network of in-
terconnecting transfer stations that make up the endocrine system,
turning hormonal secretions on and off at every site along the way.
The gradual decline in estrogen levels during the perimenopause—
which can begin as early as a woman's midthirties—disrupts this endocrine relay, producing symptoms that can range anywhere from
occasional hot flashes to debilitating psychiatric illness. I call this
phenomenon gradual estrogen deprivation syndrome, or GEDS.

In this book I will describe the biology of estrogen deprivation
and its link to the brain—why some women are so profoundly affected while others make a smooth transition through menopause.
I'll trace the hormonal journey from puberty through midlife to
demonstrate the pervasive effect of estrogen on a woman's health
and well-being at every age.

I'll share the stories of healthy, functioning, normal women who,
with no warning, slipped into hallucinatory states or suicidal depressions. Even a full barrage of antipsychotic and antidepressive
drugs could not restore these women. But estrogen could and did.
I can only wonder how many women are currently seeking psy-

chiatric help for life-threatening psychological conditions including severe depression, psychotic episodes, and suicidal impulses who are being treated with Prozac or more powerful psychoactive drugs, not realizing that their illnesses might be estrogen-related. For these women, menopause is not a "silent passage."

And I'll weave in my own story, in the chapters titled *Marcia*, because I want the women who read my book to know that I too have suffered as they have. I am not an abstract scientist or a distant clinician. I am a midlife woman who went through the darkness and emerged into the light. I want my experience to serve as a beacon for others.

As I began to write about those horrible weeks, I was sickened by the memory of my pain and humiliation. But I also felt anger. How could this have happened to me? Why didn't my doctors warn me? Why didn't I know? I knew I must tell my story, and those of others, to make women aware. To let them know they're not alone. I have a crusade, too. It is to create an atmosphere of openness and understanding so that no woman will ever have to suffer the nightmare of madness when the solution is only a blood test away.

Marcia Lawrence
March 1998

# Acknowledgments

A great many people have been extraordinarily generous in helping me to write this book, but it is Dr. Edward Klaiber who provided the foundation for understanding. This book could never have been written without his expert guidance. Whatever is of value in these pages, it is in large part owed to him for his painstaking efforts in helping me unravel the role of estrogen in mental illness. He has been unbelievably generous with his time, his devotion, and his confidence in me. His exceptional kindness and his qualities of mind and heart have engaged my deepest admiration. It has been an extraordinary privilege to work with him.

There are no words to adequately thank my psychiatrist, Dr. Ralph Wharton. It is likely that had I found my way to any other physician while in my raging psychotic state, I would either have been rushed to a psychiatric facility and given antipsychotic drugs or I would be dead. He trusted my intuitive belief that there was some physical basis for the way I was feeling, and the moment we discovered the "estrogen connection," it was Dr. Wharton who launched me on my extraordinary journey of discovery. The hallmark of his clinical skill is his uncompromising search for emotional truth pursued with humor, rigor, and tenderness. These are the qualities that have made him a deeply felt presence in the world of medicine. This book is a testament to his expert medical care.

I owe a great personal debt to Dr. Bruce McEwen and Dr. Peter Schmidt who readily responded to my many phone calls and for their generosity and patience in helping me to understand the complex mechanisms surrounding the role of estrogen. I want to thank them for sharing their information about their research, for their encouragement and genuine interest. I am also deeply indebted to many other people who have made important contributions to this book, in particular: Dr. Barbara Sherwin, Dr. Victor Henderson, Dr. Marcia Levy-Warren, Dr. Fred Naftolin, Dr. Cynthia Bethea, Dr. Ari Birkenfeld, Dr. Jean Endicott, Dr. Wilma Harrison, Dr. Andrew Herzog, Dr. Mary Collins, and Dr. Dominique Toran-Allerand.

I will be forever grateful to Dr. Clarice Kestenbaum for her skillful and compassionate intervention at a critical time in my therapy.

I want to express my heartfelt gratitude to Molly Peacock who first believed in this book. In helping me to find my voice, she enabled me to own my truth.

It has been my good fortune to have Janis Vallely as my agent, whose spirited support and sustaining belief in the message of this book, and whose perseverance through its many conceptualizations, has made this publication possible.

It was a particular pleasure to work with Catherine Whitney, an extraordinary editor and meticulous craftsman.

I am deeply grateful to the many women who have courageously shared their personal stories with me. It is their hope that describing the unique aspects of their own experience will not only be helpful to others but will advance public awareness of the complex nature of the perimenopausal transition.

I am thankful for the extraordinary support of my dear friends: Ethel Rubinstein, Dr. Sondra Gold, and Babette Rotner whose loving confrontation set me on the road to recovey. They have been an invaluable presence in my life. I am also grateful to Bernard Kaplan, principal of Great Neck North Senior High School, who has been singularly supportive. He is both a friend and colleague who shares a deep concern for all that touches the human spirit.

To my daughter, Suzanne, whose gifts of insight and generosity of heart have supported me through years of uncommon tribulation. I want to thank her for the joy she brings into my life. Her love and friendship are central to my life. I also want to pay tribute to my son, Douglas, who shared my vision of this book. His intellectual vitality, poetic sensibility, and loving heart continue to inform my life.

Finally, immeasurable gratitude to Balfour Brickner who shared every phase of work on this book. His support and encouragement, invigorating wit and wisdom, love and companionship sustained me throughout the writing of it.

Time's arrow . . . marks each moment of time
with a distinctive hand. But we cannot . . . be satisfied
with a mark to recognize each moment and a guide
to order events in temporal sequences. Uniqueness is the
essence of history, but we also crave some underlying
generality, some principles of order transcending the
distinction of moments. . . . We also need the
immanence of time's cycle.

Stephen Jay Gould
*Time's Arrow, Time's Cycle*

# 1

## *Marcia:*
## An Afternoon in August

My menopausal symptoms began around the time my husband, Ben, became ill. We had met ten years earlier, and from the very beginning there was an air of inevitability between us. He was the rabbi of a reformed temple I had joined. We felt destined to be together. At the time I was divorced and struggling to raise two young children on my own. Ben's presence provided a haven of stability and comfort. When we married, everything in my life seemed finally to settle into place.

Then Ben was diagnosed with non-Hodgkin's lymphoma. Six months after the diagnosis, he was dead.

To this day I know I'm fooling myself, but I never saw Ben's health decline. During the brief time he was ill, hope tugged at the corners of our lives. Ben was strong; it was unthinkable that such a vital man would succumb. We tried holistic cures and experimental treatments. We did everything we could to fight the disease, and never spoke of the possibility of death.

Only once did Ben allow his feeling of doom to surface. It was late at night. He had come home drained from yet another chemotherapy treatment, and we lay huddled together in our bed. Sleep no longer came easily to either of us, and we watched the lights of the George Washington Bridge flickering though our bedroom window high above the Hudson River.

Ben put his arm around my waist and gently pulled me closer to him, sliding me beneath his slightly raised body. Slowly our eyes connected, and we tried to etch that moment into memory, as if our love could somehow stay the terror of onrushing time.

Ben burrowed deeply against me, melding our bodies together. His face pressed into the hollow of my neck; then he lifted his head and brushed my cheek with his mouth.

"If I knew that we could be together forever," he whispered hoarsely, "I wouldn't take the Cytoxan." He laughed at the bitter joke of it. "What a perfect name for a drug. It's poisoning me. My life now . . ." He sighed and his lips caressed my forehead. "I love you so much," he whispered. "I know you want me to live. That's the only reason I'm going to continue this chemo. I need you to know that."

Three weeks later, Ben was dead.

In some ways the mourning process is like going blind. You learn to grope your way through the parts of your life you'd always taken for granted as a couple. Yet after Ben died there was little change in my external routine. My grief seemed to dwell in a separate space. In the two years following Ben's death, I went on with my life. Classes and students filled my days. I taught high school English in an affluent suburban community. I even completed my second book, *Acing the New SAT,* which was designed to help students increase their scores on the famous college placement exam.

During that time, I was buoyed by the support of loving friends and family. My daughter, Suzanne, and my son, Douglas, were both away at college, but they were wonderful, calling regularly and spending their school breaks with me. In spite of the ache in my heart, I was beginning to think I could live a good life without Ben.

Then I started to experience changes in my body—irregular periods, insomnia, and heart palpitations. Even though I was in my late forties, no one, not my internist or my gynecologist, ever raised the possibility that hormonal changes connected with menopause might be at the root of my problems. In retrospect, it seems absolutely unbelievable.

My gynecologist, a distinguished Park Avenue physician who'd been seeing me for many years, urged me to consult a psychiatrist just a few months before my breakdown. His timing was rather impeccable; he'd just performed a dilation and curettage (D & C) on me because of my continued menstrual irregularities, including heavy bleeding. These I now know are typical signals of the beginning of menopause. I still remember vividly how upset I was that he would even *suggest* a psychiatrist. I certainly didn't feel there was anything wrong with me mentally. In retrospect, I'm baffled that it never occurred to him to measure my estrogen levels.

My internist did no better. Although he was on the faculty of a prestigious medical school, he was unable to help me control the physical symptoms that were beginning to overwhelm me. I remember sitting in his office crying, explaining the horrible crawling sensations underneath my skin, the tingling and numbness in my fingers, the powerfully spasmodic drawing feeling deep in my groin that left me feeling both irritated and depleted.

I remember the bewildered expression in my internist's eyes when I outlined my complaints. He never even examined me. All he could say was that he'd never seen me like this before. I waited, hoping for some help, but in truth, he failed me completely. At some point I left his office. As remarkable as it now seems to me, a diagnosis was only a blood test away. Now I realize that when my doctor looked at me he saw only a traumatized, grief-stricken widow who had lost her ability to cope.

I'll never know why my doctors never considered that my condition might have had a biological basis. For I had entered perimenopause, a perilous state in which hormonal levels fluctuate widely and the supersensitive endocrine system can react badly. It is a critical time for many women, and a great number of physicians are ill-prepared to deal with their problems. In fact, although doctors may be well intentioned, as my own surely were, they often do more harm than good. In my case that was unfortunately true.

The stage had been set for my tightly wired system to snap, to cause the inevitable plunge that was to come. I learned a grave lesson: No matter how mentally acute a person is, the body can undermine both balance and perception. The body can sabotage the mind.

The summer of 1985 was my third summer without Ben. I still missed him and thought of him every day, but with time the pain of his loss had slowly receded. As I look back on that Saturday morning, the last weekend in August, I can recall no single event that would have signaled the onset of my breakdown later that day. I was spending the final days of summer at our Stockbridge house. My son, Douglas, had been accepted at Case Western Reserve University Medical School, and the preceding day he and his wife, Beth, had packed up their belongings in a rented van, pulled out of the driveway, and headed for Cleveland.

Ben had dubbed our year-round Stockbridge retreat "Woods Whole" because we were nestled in the heavily wooded Berkshire mountains of northwestern Massachusetts. We loved being there. It provided us with an opportunity for both spiritual and psychological renewal.

I felt strangely empty when I awoke on Saturday morning— as if Douglas and Beth's leaving had withdrawn some life force from the house. Yet when I examined my unsettled feelings, I thought they had less to do with my empty house than with a social engagement I had scheduled for later that afternoon. If there were a series of events that precipitated the crisis, it began with an invitation to a cocktail party.

Tanglewood concerts and predinner cocktail hours are weekend rituals in the Berkshires. They were the reason my neighbor, Roger, had come thundering into my driveway on his Harley-Davidson the week before. In his white crash helmet and protective goggles, he was hard to recognize. But as he came to a stop and pushed the goggles up against his forehead, I realized who he was. I couldn't imagine what he wanted. "Rachel and I have been trying to reach you by phone to invite you over for drinks next Saturday at four-thirty," he called out to where I was standing, leaning against the porch railing. "Since we had no luck, I decided to bike over."

I was as surprised by his invitation as I was by my acceptance. But in less time than it took for me to nod my head, Roger had revved up the motor on his bike and, with a sweeping wave of his hand, wheeled off down the driveway. At that moment, it had seemed easier to accept his invitation than to refuse. Yet I really had no interest in attending the cocktail party. I was ill at ease in his company. Roger was an intellectual sharpshooter, a heavy hitter who dominated dinner table conversations; he was consumed with self-importance. Although his cottage was slightly less than a mile down the road, under ordinary circumstances we would not have socialized.

I thought seriously about not showing up. I agonized with indecision. One day I would understand the irony. I was behaving as if my absence would be noticed, as if Roger would care one way or the other. In the end, I decided it would be rude not to go. So I chilled a bottle of wine and at 4:15 decided to walk the mile to his cottage. I thought the exercise would lift my spirits. Besides, this wasn't an occasion that warranted the degree of anxiety I was experiencing, and I felt the walk would give me a chance to unwind.

I also thought that given the distance others would be likely to travel, parking would be a problem. I was surprised, therefore, to discover when I reached Roger's driveway, that there were no cars in sight. I looked at my watch. I distinctly remembered that he had said 4:30, and it was just past that time. I climbed the steps to the screened porch and knocked.

Roger came from inside the house and opened the door with not so much warmth as interest. I remember feeling uncomfortable. I remained on the lower step. Roger stood in the doorway looking down. I glanced beyond him, my eyes spanning the length of the screened porch, which at the far end extended onto a large deck. There was a lavish spread of crackers and cheese, fruit and paté on a table along one wall and a generous assortment of wines, Perrier, and soft drinks set off as a bar in one corner.

I tried to be offhand. "I remember your saying four-thirty, Roger. Have I come on the wrong day? I don't see any cars."

His response took me by surprise. "No, the invitation was for five o'clock, not four-thirty. Rachel is in the shower. Would you mind going home and coming back in half an hour?"

"No, not at all, no problem," I said, unclear as to what had just happened. "I've been enjoying the walk anyway." I reached up to hand him the bottle of wine. "Here, keep this on ice. I'll see you in a little while."

I heard the screen door slam shut behind me as I headed down the driveway onto the main road, which would take me back home. I was hurt and humiliated. I recall thinking, *No way am I going back. I can't believe he asked me to go home and come back in half an hour. Why would he do that?* I decided I would phone Roger and say I wasn't coming.

Excuses flooded my mind. I could say that I had stepped on a piece of glass and my foot was badly cut or that my eye was injured, some foreign object flew into it. I was searching for a comfortable and reasonable excuse not to return. It never occurred to me that I didn't have to.

By the time I reached home, I felt weighted down by the crisis of indecision. Yet a part of me was adrift, as if on some inner-directed quest. I remember the feeling of being drawn to a stack of boxes high on a shelf in the living room closet. They were mostly games I had acquired over several summers from renters who had left them behind.

I instinctively reached past the familiar boxes of Monopoly and Scrabble until my hand grabbed hold of the box that said OUIJA and pulled it from the closet. I did not remember having used the Ouija board before. I didn't know how I even knew it was there, or why I had chosen it out of the pile. But that spontaneous act was to be the defining moment which precipitated my plunge into madness.

I lifted the laminated board out of its case. Then, casually carrying it to the far end of the room, I set the board down on one end of the dining room table, a solid slab of deep-textured green and black marble, the dominant center of my memories with Ben.

Sitting in the presence of the board, I felt high-spirited. Slowly I set the triangular pointer down and gently, though with some firmness, moved it along the two rows of the alphabet.

I remember joking with Ben about my present state of affairs, barely aware that I was sliding the pointer up and down on the board.

"Well, Ben, I have about ten minutes left before I have to call Roger. Tell me, how is lying treated in the spirit world?"

I felt a surge of movement in the pointer. It seemed suddenly to have become lighter under my touch. A rush of almost electric intensity flowed through me. My heart began pounding furiously. My breathing quickened. I could barely form the words "Ben, is that you?"

With one flash of motion, the pointer flew up to the word YES, located in one corner of the board. I was stunned, then elated.

"I can't believe this is happening, Ben. This is wonderful."

Suddenly the pointer began to shift in all directions, sliding from letter to letter until it stopped. It was as though I could feel Ben's hand on top of mine. I shivered with delight. It had spelled out the word SURPRISE.

"This is a wonderful surprise. It's unbelievable." Then, half-speaking to myself, I said, "This is so perfect. I could really use your help right now. I have about ten minutes left before I have to call Roger to tell him I'm not returning. But I'm really not sure what reason to give. I'm open for suggestions."

Slowly and deliberately, in what seems to me even to this day utterly incomprehensible, the pointer beneath my hand moved across the board and spelled out the word PRAY.

I have thought about his word for a long time, and there is no way, even now, that in my conscious mind I can find a rationale, or a clue of any kind, that would have summoned this response from my unconscious. I was not a person who believed in prayer as a solution. Although I had been married to a rabbi, we were not what one would describe as religious, and in many ways I viewed Ben's religious duties as a thing apart from our lives. Ben would often say, "I am not God's holy emissary. I have no holy water to pour over you. *Rabbi* means teacher. That's all I am." But he was far, far more. He had been a highly creative and spiritual man who possessed none of the trappings of dogma or parochialism.

"Are you serious, Ben? You want me to pray? Like 'The Lord is my shepherd'—that kind of prayer?"

The pointer shifted rapidly under my hand, pausing long enough for me to read each letter. I laughed out loud. Ben had spelled the word PEDESTRIAN.

"You want me to find something more original?" I asked gleefully.

The pointer flew up to YES. "Are you telling me if I pray, I will find what I need to say to Roger?"

The pointer shifted with great speed in a series of convoluted movements around the board, then slid back to YES.

It seemed outrageous and improbable that by randomly choosing a passage from the Bible, I would be handed a resolution to the Roger affair, but at this point I trusted what I was receiving from the board. I felt calm and centered. I felt that I was in Ben's presence. I would pray.

The structure of my Stockbridge home is unusual in two aspects. It is six-sided, with sliding glass doors that lead to a wraparound deck, and the living room, dining room, and kitchen are upstairs while the bedrooms and study are on the ground floor. They are connected by a spiral staircase. We always kept the two volumes of the Bible in the downstairs study. Though I was still skeptical, as I made my way down the stairs, I spoke to Ben.

"You know I'm a bit of a doubting Thomas, Ben. But if you want me to pray, I'm going to give it a try."

I took the two-volume set of the Bible off the top shelf of the bookcase and sat down. I had no idea where to begin.

I also had no sense that Ben was with me. I was fainthearted about this enterprise. Part of me wondered if it were all some imagined happening. But I had said I would pray, and if I were in Ben's presence, that was what I would do. Besides, I thought, smiling to myself, he had promised me an answer, although judging from what I held in my hands, it hardly seemed likely that I would find one.

I looked through the pages in Volume 1. Then I put it aside.

Genesis and Exodus didn't seem to lend themselves to prayer. "If it's all right with you, Ben, I'm going to read from Volume Two," I announced. "I think I'll read from the Psalms." They were closer to my idea of prayer. Then, quite spontaneously and for no reason I can recall, I said, "No, I've decided to read from Proverbs instead. I've never read them before."

I read slowly through the thirty-three verses in Chapter 1, and then I said in an effort to reassure Ben of my sincerity, "I really am trying to read them with a full heart." Then I announced, "I'm going on to Chapter Two now," and read through the twenty-two verses in Chapter 2.

I was aware that it was getting late and I was starting to become anxious. Halfway through chapter 3, I stopped reading. "It's after five o'clock, Ben. I have to phone Roger. If you have some message for me, I hope it's soon."

It was. When I reached Proverbs 3:28, what felt like an electric current surged through my body. It read,

*Say not unto thy neighbor, Go, and come again,*
*and tomorrow I will give; when thou has it by thee.*

Out of more then two thousand pages that constitute the two volumes of the Hebrew Bible, I had found my answer. I never did call Roger. Instead, I raced back upstairs to the board, crying and laughing at the same time. I no longer had to move the pointer. It swept along under its own power with the barest touch of my finger. "I love you, Ben," I said. "Thank you." And Ben wrote, THIS HAS BEEN GOD'S GIFT TO YOU. NOW WE CAN WORK TOGETHER. With that message, I felt suffused in a glow of love and warmth. At that moment, I slipped the bounds of reality and surrendered myself to another world.

I don't remember how long I stayed with the board. It had to have been several hours. I recall that at some point the room grew dark and I had to get up and turn on the overhead track lights. I found it difficult to disengage from the board. It was like putting down the receiver of a phone and walking away from a lover's conversation.

I apologized to Ben for the interruption but explained that I had not been able to see the letters on the board. Then I realized he would have known that; he was now a part of my consciousness. I felt as if our minds had fused and I was filled with his presence.

It suddenly occurred to me that all the time I thought I needed to follow the letters on the board to understand the message, I was in fact hearing them, not reading them. And while I would continue to feel the need to use the Ouija board, I would *hear* the message long before it was fully spelled out.

The voice began near my right temple. It was not even a voice really, but an impression, then a whisper that gradually became louder and more insistent. It was a voice that, in a matter of days, would become a compelling authority controlling each detail of my life. First Ben, speaking for God, and then God Himself, would become the core around which the hallucinated voice was structured.

When I returned to the board, I expressed my fatigue. "I'm exhausted, Ben. Full of love, but exhausted." The intensity of the emotion and the concentration I had expended trying to decode the messages on the board had thoroughly drained me.

Yet tired as I was, I was alert to the fact that the pointer had noticeably slowed. I sensed, intuitively, that something was wrong. "What is it, Ben? What's going on? I have a feeling there's something you want to tell me." The pointer moved as though with some hesitancy. It still slid easily around the board, but I felt a change in the way Ben was communicating with me. My sense of him was somehow distanced, his words less intimate, less loving, and it was the first time I experienced fear.

MARCIA, WHAT I SAID TO YOU IS TRUE. GOD HAS GIVEN YOU HIS BLESSING AND HE DOES WANT US TO WORK TOGETHER. BUT THERE IS A REASON. HE HAS CHOSEN YOU BECAUSE HE FEELS YOU ARE THE ONLY ONE WHO CAN PREVENT A SITUATION THAT, AT THIS MOMENT, HAS THE POTENTIAL FOR BRINGING ABOUT THE MOST CATASTROPHIC CONSEQUENCES.

In spite of the fact that we had been conversing through the board for the past several hours, it was the first time Ben had addressed me by my name. For some reason, this formality had a chilling effect. When Ben spelled out my name, I experienced what was to be for the next two-and-a-half weeks a prelude to fear, not love, for my name would become the harbinger of messages that would steal my will and dignity.

"But God can do anything, Ben. What is it He wants? You know I will do it, but I don't understand."

The pointer seemed to move with a more definite purpose.

IT'S NOT THAT SIMPLE. BEFORE HE CAN REVEAL TO YOU THE NATURE OF THE TASK YOU WILL UNDERTAKE, THERE ARE SOME TESTS YOU MUST PASS TO PROVE YOUR SENSE OF COMMITMENT AND WORTH. THERE ARE NOT MANY PEOPLE HE WOULD CALL UPON.

I felt uplifted, blessed, and then felt humility and wonder at being chosen. All feelings of fatigue disappeared. I was eager to help. "Just tell me what He wants me to do."

I realized that whatever Ben was about to ask on God's behalf, there would be little ground for appeal or negotiation. It was a strange request. Ben said I was to memorize a page in Volume 1 of the Bible. I would know the page when I came to it. I was to have it learned within three days. Then he could tell me in what way I, alone, was chosen to help God.

As I write, I am stunned by the ease with which a mind can collapse. I find it incredible that I would spend the next three days memorizing commandments 18 through 32 given by the Lord to Moses and Aaron in Leviticus 15. I couldn't imagine why I was asked to memorize that particular segment, dealing with the procedures that are required when an Israelite male or female experiences discharges from the sexual organs. The specific verses focus on menstruation, laws concerning sexual relations with women who are menstruating, and laws designating the rituals for purification. Now, of course, I'm sure that some part of my unconscious mind was struggling to alert me to the biological changes in my body. And the drama I played out in this critical phase of my breakdown was weighted with religious rituals. Only a few short days from the time I was charged with memorizing the commandments from Leviticus, I was performing commanded acts of an intensely sexual and autoerotic nature.

During the next three days I barely slept, and I ate very little. I found Ben's voice gradually receding, replaced by God's, and I was locked in the prison of His commands. On the one hand, I concentrated on memorizing the passages, yet on the other hand, I was weakly fighting against the powerful force that held me captive.

As I repeated the commandments over and over, I would feel pressure, like a giant mass, expanding deep inside me. Then it would recede in strong and even movement, my body frozen into a corner of the couch. There were times I tried to produce the sensation on my own, to prove to myself that it was only my unconscious. I willed it to happen. But no matter how hard I concentrated, my body remained dormant. Yet once the small eruptions beyond my will began to mushroom, I was helpless to stop them.

The Ouija board was constantly at my side. I was becoming more distracted, gradually disconnecting from the real world, which no longer held my interest. It was a macabre perversion. I turned to what I must have believed was some form of spiritual refuge, yielding myself up to the exquisite promise of another world, which instead was soon to threaten my existence. No one could have convinced me then that the voices in my head, or the spontaneous upheavals in my body, were not the results of powerful supernatural forces. Deluded by intimations of conscious survival, I entered a kind of spiritual autism.

It was as if I were in an auto race, caught in the air slip of the car ahead, being pulled along, floating within a vehicle that I was not driving. Part of me was struggling with the verses in Leviticus. They were difficult to memorize; they all seemed to be variations on the same theme—discharges, menstrual impurities, rituals for purification. Yet all these were to become a grist for my unconscious.

Today I turn the pages in the Bible and glance over the hundreds of other more innocuous, even more spiritual possibilities. I ask myself whether my being ordered to read a "random" page from the Book of Leviticus was influenced by a guiding intelligence that had impressed this design on me from the beginning or whether, in some phenomenal leap, my unconscious mind had already made the hormonal connection. The Ouija board was at once the instrument that precipitated my episode and the tool that enabled me to keep my boundaries firm. Had everything remained encased within my psyche without an external object with which to interact, I may not have had a concrete symbol to finally throw away. The Ouija board became the symbol of a soul at war with itself. In time, it allowed my unconscious to rescue me from myself by ordering me to destroy it.

I had surrendered to a delusionary world. I was no longer capable of understanding the difference between my fantastic inner life and my outer reality. Had I understood the biology of menopause, I might have recognized my early symptoms and prevented such a catastrophic happening. I would have understood the biochemical mechanisms that not only had altered my hormonal balance but were destroying the integrity of my mind. Instead, I was swept along on a furious tide whose destination remained mysterious and frightening.

# 2

# The Hormonal Battleground

I was quickly soaring away from reality. I often wonder now what might have happened if someone I trusted had said to me at the beginning of it all, "Marcia, this is not real." I don't think I would have believed him. And if anyone had suggested that my delusions were triggered by a mundane biological event, I would have thought her insane. Although I was educated, well-read, and medically aware, I had never heard that a hormonal imbalance could wreak such havoc on the brain.

However, in the years since my breakdown, I have made this research an important focus of my life. I have taken on the task of sifting through the contradictory opinions of scientists, medical researchers, and physicians to clear a path to the truth about menopause. It has been frustrating and often disturbing work. I realized early on that talking about estrogen meant walking through a minefield of debate. I also saw that in spite of the growing documentation of a link between estrogen deficiency and mental illness, many doctors refuse even to acknowledge the possibility. Perhaps this is because medical specialties have become too tightly compartmentalized. It can be threatening for gynecologists to hand over a piece of their territory to endocrinologists and psychiatrists. Likewise, there are a lot of mental health professionals who resist the idea that certain psychoses may be best treated by gynecologists and endocrinologists. It was much easier for everybody when any discussion of estrogen was joined to the topic of fertility.

But it is growing harder to compartmentalize estrogen because we now know that there are estrogen receptors in nearly every part of the body. Obviously, problems related to these receptor sites can involve many medical specialties. In recent years we've seen tremendous publicity about findings that connect estrogen depletion to increased incidences of heart disease and osteoporosis in postmenopausal women. But the effects of low estrogen levels are much more insidious, and they begin much earlier than was previously thought.

In the past menopause was viewed as a discrete event—the cessation of menses. Now we understand that menopause is a *process* that takes place over a period of years. While it typically occurs between the ages of forty-seven and fifty-five, it can begin as early as a woman's mid-thirties. The exact time frame varies among women. We call this period the *perimenopause*, meaning, literally, "around menopause." During the perimenopause, production of estrogen and progesterone, the two female hormones, begins to decline. This process can cause any number of uncomfortable symptoms, such as hot flashes, sleeplessness, heart palpitations, vaginal dryness, lessened libido, and mood swings. For some women, the symptoms are barely noticeable. Others suffer a great deal. And, since there are estrogen receptors in the brain, about 15 percent of women are beset by serious psychiatric illness when estrogen levels are depleted. These uniquely susceptible women may lapse into severe depression, or, as I did, they may disassociate from reality, with psychotic symptoms. Studies support the conclusion that this condition, which I call gradual estrogen deprivation syndrome, or GEDS, occurs primarily in the perimenopause— often before any visible physical symptoms of menopause occur.

During the five or six years before a woman's last menstrual period, hormonal levels can fluctuate widely. These fluctuations disrupt the brain's neurotransmitters, which send and receive messages that control all our bodily functions. As a result, the complex wiring in the brain seems to become tangled. Tangled wiring is a perfect image for the feelings many women report, as they are suddenly and inexplicably torn away from their sense of normalcy and well-being.

Some women's brains are exquisitely sensitive to even the slightest alteration in chemical balance. A vast array of puzzling symptoms can result from even a small or gradual hormonal shift. It is not possible to pinpoint a universal response to estrogen deprivation. Everyone is unique; all of us are "wired" just a little differently.

## The Invisible Perimenopause

One reason that GEDS often goes undiagnosed is that nobody's looking for it. Many of the women I interviewed began experiencing disturbing symptoms before they hit their mid-forties and while they were still menstruating. Even their gynecologists didn't consider menopause—especially when their symptoms appeared psychological. Yet research has shown that years before a woman may have any idea she is beginning to experience perimenopause, real physical changes are occurring. PET scans, for example, show definite changes in the blood flow during perimenopause, which can account for loss of mental acuity. Other studies on the effects of estrogen reduction during that time reveal that a distinct estrogen drop-off before a woman enters menopause causes a loss in bone density.

Laura, a public school teacher I interviewed, was only forty-four when she was suddenly beset by episodes of extreme dizziness. She recalls being at school and finding it hard to maintain her equilibrium. "It would be time for lunch and I would wonder if I could make it from my classroom to the cafeteria. I can remember almost getting there and feeling like I was going to fall on the floor and faint dead away. It was terrifying."

When Laura went to her gynecologist, he promptly dismissed the idea that her sudden vertigo might be related to menopause, noting that she was far too young to be experiencing any of the symptoms. His "off the top of my head" diagnosis was stress. Laura believed him, since she was still having normal periods.

But then Laura began to have anxiety attacks, and she became very frightened. "One Sunday I was driving to a nearby garden center, which is something I love to do. I remember finding a parking space, pulling in, and getting out of the car. It was a beautiful, sunny day, and as usual the garden center was mobbed. I got as far as the split railing fence when I suddenly began to feel a pounding in my chest; my heart was beating very fast. I didn't think I was having a heart attack, but I broke out in a cold sweat and became nauseated. I couldn't move. I leaned on the fence for a few minutes, and finally was able to get back in the car. I sat there for about fifteen minutes trying to get control of myself. I felt alternately like I was going to just come out of my skin and like I was going to shrink back so far inside myself that I'd never come out again. It was a horrible feeling. I was finally able to compose myself enough to drive home. And that was only the first time. It got so bad that I couldn't control it.

"I had to find out what was wrong with me. I went to every kind of doctor. I went to eye, ear, and nose people, heart people, and no one had answers. At one point I became convinced that I had a brain tumor, but when that was eliminated I thought I was crazy. Yet through it all I kept going to work, even though it was a terrifying ordeal. I recall one incident in a classroom. All the children were in groups, and I was moving around from one group to another when suddenly I felt that by now familiar wave of anxiety sweep over me. I fought down a total panic attack. I can still remember how the children were staring at me. It was like I was totally dysfunctional. I couldn't think about anything. I couldn't concentrate. I felt as if I needed to get out from where I was, yet I didn't know where I was going to go."

Laura finally ended up in therapy, but this only increased her frustration. Her therapist refused to acknowledge the physical aspects of what was happening to her. He felt that she had just come to a vulnerable place in her life. Laura was forced to suffer from her debilitating symptoms until she began to display more conventional symptoms of menopause—such as hot flashes and irregular periods. Finally, to alleviate those symptoms, her doctor put her on estrogen.

"With estrogen replacement I felt like my old self again," Laura says. "It was miraculous. My hot flashes were gone. I regained my energy. The panic attacks, the terrible anxiety, and the severe depression disappeared almost overnight. It was just unbelievable. I thought I'd gone crazy."

Laura's GEDS was never recognized, even though there is now substantial data to support the effects of gradual estrogen deprivation. It is scandalous that women are being asked to present visible evidence—such as hot flashes and the complete cessation of menses—before doctors will consider the validity of their menopausal symptoms.

## Entering the Minefield

I once naively assumed that science operated on an objective scale—devoid of political agendas, personal biases, and hyperemotional overtones. I've certainly learned differently while researching the role of estrogen in women's lives. Perhaps no other medical issue today is as fraught with so much emotional baggage and so many opposing positions. Menopause has become the new empowerment zone for feminism. "Fabulous at fifty" is the clarion call. No one is interested in talking about the women who *don't* feel so fabulous. In certain circles a woman like myself, who dares to suggest that menopause makes some women "sick," is considered a traitor to her sex.

"Some feminist leaders who have previously spoken out for women's issues tend to trivialize the impact of menopause, and accuse those women who complain of negative experiences of being afraid to face the reality of aging," observed Dr. Elizabeth Vliet, author of *Screaming to Be Heard,* which details how difficult it is for women to get their medical complaints addressed. In her book, Dr. Vliet recounts overhearing one feminist activist describe her menopause in this fashion: "I think it lasted about an hour. I don't see what the fuss is all about." This dismissive and politically correct view of menopause makes it very hard for legitimate medical information to be accepted.

The irony of this position is clear. When women won't acknowledge that they're having problems because they fear a societal backlash, they don't get treatment and they actually *do* become ill. We can be grateful that some highly visible feminists are beginning to break the silence. Patricia Ireland, president of the National Organization for Women, has admitted suffering cognitive lapses before she began hormone replacement therapy. The author Letty Cottin Pogrebin wrote about her own mental pain in her 1996 book *Getting Over Getting Older*. Anna Quindlen wrote in a *New York Times* column that "when I began to wake bolt upright in the middle of the night and start forgetting the names of my children, I initially thought I was losing my mind." It is a form of courage of these prominent women to speak out—to bring the truth into the open. But the debate still rages.

The hot button of the debate is whether menopause is "natural." As one female endocrinologist bluntly told me when I spoke to her about my book, "You're going to get slapped down on this issue. You're going to get a lot of backlash. I've experienced it myself. There's an entire movement that is fiercely dedicated to the message that menopause is a 'natural' biological event and we doctors are trying to medicalize it by shoving hormones down everybody's throat." This same doctor was thoughtful in her response to the question of whether or not menopause should be considered an illness. "I don't know," she replied. "You have symptoms caused by a biological event. Pregnancy also causes symptoms, but we don't call it an illness because it's a natural event. The question should be whether we view menopause as a natural event. The fact that women's life spans have increased tremendously means that the ball game has changed, and we may want to handle our approach to menopause differently."

Clearly, women's medical issues are vastly different than they were 125 years ago, when the average woman's life span was around fifty years. Since most women didn't survive beyond menopause, how can we compare their experience with ours? For most women today, menopause occurs at *midlife,* not the end of life. Our average life expectancies are approaching 80 years. So while most people consider menopause a "natural" life experience, the evidence seems to point in just the opposite direction—that menopause is, if anything, an *unnatural* life experience. It is medical technology, not nature, that has increased our longevity. Why are we so opposed to using medical technology when it comes to menopause? Surely if Mother Nature had intended menopause to be a natural life event, she would have intervened with some marvelous hormonal overdrive to accommodate it. It is perfectly legitimate to raise questions and investigate the experience of menopause as one would a disease.

## Menopause as a Deficiency Disease

"A disease is a state that harms a person's body, and menopause certainly does this," says Dr. Geoffrey Redmond, author of *A Woman's Hormones.* "Unlike most diseases, this happens to have an incidence of occurrence in one hundred percent of the female population. The cause is depletion of follicles in the ovary; its symptoms are those of the resulting lack of estrogen. Therefore, menopause is an endocrine-deficiency disease. Some women are comforted if they can think of menopause as natural. Of course it is, in the sense that it is inevitable, but not in the sense that nothing needs to be done about it."

This makes perfect medical sense. Still, the detractors are outspoken and highly visible. Dr. Wulf Utian is a professor of reproductive biology at Case Western Reserve University. He founded the North American Menopause Society in 1989 and is now president of its international counterpart. Dr. Utian is offended by the very idea of menopause being considered a disease. He speaks as if he must defend the "honor" of menopause. "Menopause is getting a bad rap," Dr. Utian complains. "It's being cast as a disease and built into an industry. There is very little evidence that the biological process of going through menopause means any real change in emotional or cognitive functioning."

Dr. Alice Rossi, of the Social and Demographic Research Institute at the University of Massachusetts at Amherst, goes even further, dismissing the menopause issue altogether. "Estrogen," she declares, "is a therapy in search of a disease."

Such a claim seems outrageous in the face of the evidence as we know it. It is now widely acknowledged that estrogen loss in women lessens bone density, substantially increases the risk of heart disease, and can impair cognitive functioning. How can anyone say that a condition that yields itself to organic treatment is not a disease? The notion of a disease points to a physical cause, and in the case of menopause medication can actually reverse the physical symptoms. This concept shifts our whole view of menopause into the field of endocrinopathy. And some experts believe this is exactly what we *should* be doing.

Dr. Edward Klaiber is a reproductive endocrinologist and research scientist at the Worcester State Hospital in Massachusetts. Dr. Klaiber has been conducting clinical studies on the relationship between female hormones and bodily systems for more than thirty years. Long before others had even considered the possibility, he was exploring the effects of hormones on the brain. In a significant five-year double-blind study that tracked the effects of estrogen depletion on psychological illness, Dr. Klaiber and his colleagues, Drs. Donald Broverman and William Vogel of the Worcester State Hospital, studied forty severely depressed women, both menopausal and nonmenopausal. Some of these women had been in Worcester State Hospital for as long as nine years. They had been on three or four different antidepressants and had undergone electric shock therapy, but nothing worked. Dr. Klaiber gave twenty-three of the women high doses of estrogen while seventeen other women received a placebo. The results were impressive. The women treated with estrogen improved dramatically, while those given the placebo showed no significant change.

Recent studies suggest that estrogen may be the key by which menopausal psychiatric illness can be diagnosed as a distinct physical condition, not unlike the symptoms experienced in premenstrual syndrome and postpartum psychiatric illness. "There are many triggers in the female depressives that we studied," says Dr. Klaiber, "but each one of these situations can clearly be related to a hormonal situation. There has been either an estrogen deficiency or a component of endocrine effect which blocks the action and effect of estrogen."

Today Dr. Klaiber's studies are widely regarded as the seminal work in this field. He has also generously given his time to serve as a resource for my work. He states that "menopause is an estrogen deficiency illness. The idea that menopause does not predispose women to illness is nonsense, because the largest number of deaths in menopausal women are from heart attacks. Four hundred thousand women a year die from heart attacks, and if that's not an illness, I don't know what is."

## The Medical Consequences of Estrogen Depletion

Let's examine some of the known effects of estrogen deprivation common in women after menopause. The two most pronounced, and most deadly, are heart disease and osteoporosis.

Heart disease is the *number-one* killer of women after menopause, although it is relatively rare before menopause, except for women who have had premenopausal hysterectomies. Scientists believe that estrogen is the factor that makes the difference, although they are not certain why. It appears, however, that estrogen increases the levels of high-density lipoprotein (or HDL, the "good cholesterol") and decreases the levels of low-density lipoprotein (or LDL, the "bad cholesterol"). HDL cholesterol has a protective influence on the arteries, guarding against the buildup of fatty deposits on the artery walls. Estrogen also appears to increase dilation of the blood vessels, making them less likely to spasm.

The heart disease–estrogen connection is now widely ac-

cepted after rigorous clinical trials. One of the most famous, released in 1989, was conducted by Dr. Trudy L. Bush and her colleagues at the National Institutes of Health's Heart, Lung, and
Blood Institute. It placed 2,269 women, between the ages of
forty and sixty-nine on estrogen replacement therapy or a
placebo and followed them for five years. The death rate among
the women taking estrogen was only one-third that of those
who were taking the placebo.

A more recent study, published in the January 18, 1995, issue
of the *Journal of the American Medical Association,* was conducted over three years at seven medical centers in the United
States. In the study, 875 healthy women between the ages of
forty-five and sixty-four were placed on one of three regimens.
The first was unopposed estrogen replacement therapy, and the
other two used different combinations, including progestin. The
results showed that estrogen alone had the greatest effect on
preventing heart disease.

Studies are ongoing that will increase our understanding of
the estrogen–heart disease mechanism. Of course, there are
many issues surrounding the use of estrogen replacement therapy, such as the potential increased risk of breast and endometrial cancers. I'll address those issues in chapter 9. However,
concerns about cancer do not negate the fact that estrogen is a
critical factor in preventing heart disease.

The second major effect of estrogen depletion is osteoporosis. According to the Johns Hopkins medical letter, *Health After
50,* a recent Gallup poll found that American women know
dangerously little about the risk of osteoporosis. The survey
showed that more than 80 percent of those polled did not recognize the link between osteoporosis and the one million bone

fractures it causes every year. And fewer than 10 percent thought osteoporosis was life threatening, even though some 50,000 deaths can be attributed to it annually, usually as a result of complications in the aftermath of a fall. Half of those at high risk for the disease thought it was unlikely they would ever be affected; nearly 75 percent at high risk had never discussed the condition with their doctors.

These are startling statistics. Even the American College of Obstetricians and Gynecologists acknowledges that osteoporosis is second only to heart disease as the greatest health hazard associated with menopause.

The risk of osteoporosis differs among women, according to heredity, diet, exercise, and other factors. Women with larger, denser bones tend to be less susceptible than women with smaller more fragile makeups. Since calcium is the mineral mostly responsible for building and maintaining bone strength, women with problems absorbing calcium, or lactose intolerant women, may be at greater risk.

Many women believe, and are told, that the best way to prevent osteoporosis is to take in enough calcium, through food or supplements. Calcium intake is important. However, it is now known that estrogen is the key to making sure that calcium is absorbed and utilized properly. Hormone replacement therapy is now commonly recommended for the prevention and treatment of osteoporosis.

Recently two major drug companies have been running clinical trials on osteoporosis drugs, and early results indicate that they may be highly effective. However, it would be a step backward if women began taking osteoporosis drugs instead of hormone replacement therapy. The systemic effects of estrogen cannot be matched with targeted treatments. For example, the decline of female hormones also has an impact on other hormonal systems—most prominently the thyroid. For women with a susceptibility to thyroid imbalances, estrogen depletion can trigger a severe onset of the disease.

According to Dr. Elizabeth Vliet, thyroid disorders in women which "often cause disturbances in mood and menstrual cycles, worsening PMS, atypical depression, excessive fatigue, and anxiety syndromes are often given a psychiatric label. What often happens is that only the thyroid hormones are checked, without looking at the brain hormone SFH, which is a much more sensitive indicator of excessive or declining thyroid."

Michele is a case in point. "I always had a minor thyroid problem," she told me. She recalled how it had emerged during her freshman year in college. She managed to push it out of her mind, and so did her parents. "I remember going home from college feeling exhausted. I also had a lot of hair loss, and I can recall my parents commenting on my slightly swollen neck. But they attributed everything to the stress of college, studying too hard, keeping late hours. There were no other symptoms to indicate that there was anything wrong with me. Every doctor I went to would routinely touch my neck and say, "Oh, we should look at that." I had all the standard blood tests, and no one ever picked it up. Even my periods were fine."

Then, when she was forty-two, several traumatic events converged in Michele's life. A crisis with her job as a high-profile executive, the onset of her perimenopause, and a worsening of her thyroid condition united like a tidal wave to destroy her ability to cope. "It was like spinning down into a vortex," she said. "Spinning, falling, flipping, over and over. Every single thing in my life came totally undone. It was the first and only time in my life when stress from job trauma triggered personal feelings of betrayal, of loss and abandonment. But all these feelings were so wildly extreme and magnified. I think it must have been at that point that I suffered a total endocrine system breakdown."

Since the thyroid is a component of the endocrine system, it participates in the cascade of chemical reactions precipitated once the hormonal imbalance of perimenopause is triggered. In fact, research suggests that Michele's form of thyroid disorder, called Hashimoto's disease, presents itself in women around the age of fifty, close enough to Michele's age to fit her profile. But it was the enormous stress she was facing in her work life that tipped the balance.

Blood tests revealed a dramatic imbalance in the rates that Michele's estrogen and progesterone were dropping. While her estrogen level was just beginning to decline, her progesterone was diminishing much faster. The high level of estrogen and the low level of progesterone triggered symptoms so frightening that Michele said, "I don't even know how to describe them. When things were at their absolute worst, I was getting my period every nineteen days, and it was so profuse that I was unable to leave my apartment or schedule appointments for the first two days. To top it all off, on the day before my period I would go into a fit of convulsive shaking, terrible chills and shivering, and I couldn't move or eat, almost like I was in some kind of comatose state.

"When I told my gynecologist, she said, 'I don't know anything about that. I've never heard of that.' But months later, when I described my symptoms to an endocrinologist, he said, 'This happens right before your period? It sounds to me like it's a severe deficit of progesterone.'" Michele's consternation at her gynecologist's inadequacy was overshadowed by her obvious relief in having a diagnosis. "I'm finally on thyroid medication," she said, "which should stabilize me, but I'm also taking a birth control pill, just as an interim thing, until my period is more under control."

Michele's symptoms were caught early by an alert endocrinologist. But her experience shows that physicians even compartmentalize the endocrine system—truly amazing when you consider the interactions of hormones in the body.

A recent scientific discovery might finally get the attention of the medical community and force it to acknowledge the pervasive role of estrogen. Scientists have identified a previously unknown estrogen receptor whose influence spreads to virtually every bodily system. This beta receptor has been found in organs that previously were thought to have no relationship to estrogen—such as the liver, intestines, bladder, kidneys, and lungs. It has also been found in the blood vessels. Now scientists are beginning to ask: Is there any part of the body that is *not* affected by estrogen?

If we know that estrogen is ubiquitous in our cellular functions, why is the medical community so reluctant to take the obvious next step—acknowledging estrogen's role in brain activity?

## The Path to the Brain

"Our understanding of the mechanisms of the brain is still in its infancy," says the neurobiologist Dr. Richard Restak, "but in the field of neuroscience the search is under way for some fundamental organizing principle, a neurobiological unified field theory, that will unite observable human behavior with the action of molecules operating at levels far below our current ability to observe."

This statement is provocative. Might that organizing principle be related to hormones? What we so far understand is that the brain is composed of vast bundles of highly organized and interconnective nerve fibers responding to electrochemical charges. These charges create and fire off an endless stream of information and direction to every cell of our bodies. Imagine this: An electrical impulse flashes across the axon of a nerve cell, a neuron. It then encounters a canyon between the neuron cells, called a synapse. It needs a ride; it can't breach the canyon by itself. Instantaneously a chemical transporter (called a neurotransmitter) appears, allowing the electrical impulse to continue its lightning trip across the synapse to the next neuron. This is repeated endlessly. Without the action of the neurotransmitter, the electrical impulse to the brain is stranded.

Receptors, the proteins in and on brain cells that receive chemical messages and dictate what those brain cells do, respond directly to this complex world of chemicals. Any alteration in the balance of these receptors and their chemical transmitters directly affects what occurs on the chemical and molecular levels. Of course, any change could be expected to affect thoughts and feelings on the behavioral level.

The four most vital neurotransmitters in relation to hormones are acetylcholine, dopamine, norepinephrine, and serotonin. In various combinations, too little or too much of these neurotransmitters can affect concentration, memory, libido, mood, sleep cycles, and appetite. There's broad agreement among psychiatrists that neurotransmitters are the key to certain behaviors—not just psychiatric behaviors, like schizophrenia or bipolar illness, but ordinary behaviors as well. Our thought processes, our concentration levels, our moods and sleep patterns; all involve the action of neurotransmitters. If the neurotransmitters aren't functioning properly, obviously our mental and emotional processes will be affected—sometimes severely.

What does this have to do with estrogen?

Dr. Klaiber's research has allowed him to understand this connection better than most. A major part of his work over the past thirty years has been devoted to studying the effects of hormones on the brain. In the beginning, the very idea was dismissed in medical journals. It was believed that there was a "blood-brain barrier"—that is, hormones in the blood had no mechanism by which to enter the brain.

This theory was disproved when researchers using radioactive-labeled tracers injected estrogen into the blood. As much as 20 percent of the injected estrogen could subsequently be detected in the brain.

In his studies at Worcester State Hospital, Dr. Klaiber has found a direct link between estrogen and the production and breakdown of neurotransmitters. He has reached the conclusion that estrogen increases the production of norepinephrine and serotonin, as well as prevents their metabolism, or inactivation.

In addition, estrogen seems to affect blood flow to the brain. Using a sophisticated scanning technique called SPECT (single photon emission computed tomography), Dr. Klaiber and his colleagues were able to observe decreased blood flow to the brain in menopausal women with low estrogen levels. Once they were treated with estrogen, these women showed measurably improved blood flow to the brain.

Recently there has been tremendous excitement in medical circles about studies showing that estrogen may help prevent or diminish the effects of Alzheimer's disease and dementia in the elderly. It is possible that the ultimate understanding of estrogen and the brain may come as a result of these studies.

Here's the theory: There are many receptor sites for estrogen in the brain, especially in the hippocampus, where much of our memory function is localized. The hippocampus seems to need estrogen to maintain healthy connections to other parts of the brain. Research conducted by Dr. Bruce McEwen of the Laboratory of Neuroendocrinology at New York City's Rockefeller University has shown that estrogen increases the number of connections between nerve cells in the hippocampus. "Estrogen spurs an important memory enzyme," Dr. McEwen explains. "This enzyme, called choline acetyltransferase, is a brain chemical which is abnormally low in Alzheimer's patients." Acetyltransferase is needed to synthesize the neurotransmitter acetylcholine. Dr. McEwen believes enzyme deficiency could explain some of the forgetfulness, cognitive impairments, and psychosis associated with Alzheimer's disease—and more important, lack of estrogen could be one reason choline acetyltransferase levels fall. Dr. McEwen's tests with laboratory animals have shown that estrogen deprivation actually decreases the number of synaptic connections, but these connections are remade within a few days after estrogen is administered. "We know that estrogen influences the architecture of the brain in neural development, and that Alzheimer's is a disease of brain death," explains Dr. Dominique Toran-Allerand. "But most people are not aware that the brain is a major target of estrogen."

Perhaps the most compelling evidence to link estrogen deprivation with Alzheimer's disease came out of Dr. Barbara Sherwin's work with Lupron, a hormone often used to shrink benign tumors. Since tumors in women's reproductive organs are estrogen dependent, the Lupron, which overstimulates both the pituitary and the ovary so they no longer manufacture estrogen, was given to patients to shut down their ovaries. This allowed benign tumors to shrink so they could be more easily removed surgically.

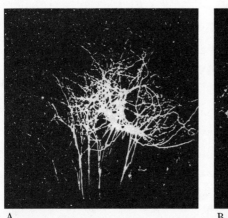 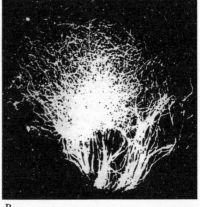

A                                                    B

A dramatic example of the effect of added estrogen on the brain. An embryonic nerve fiber from the part of a rat's brain involved in reproduction (photo A) sprouted many new wiring connections after exposure to estrogen (photo B). Photos by Dr. D. Toran-Allerand. Reprinted by permission of *Brain Research*.

Dr. Sherwin, a professor of psychology and OB–GYN at McGill University in Montreal, found that Lupron worked very well at shrinking the tumors, but she discovered some surprising side effects. Her study showed that the women treated with Lupron—thus halting their estrogen production—experienced measurable cognitive deficits, most notably memory loss. When Lupron treatment was reversed and estrogen was given, the women's memories improved.

Dr. Victor Henderson, who is a professor in the Department of Neurology and head of the Division of Cognitive Neuroscience and the Neurogerontology at the University of Southern California, studied 2,418 women and found that those on hormone replacement therapy were 40 percent less likely to develop Alzheimer's disease. His study, titled "The Role of Estrogen Replacement Therapy in Older Women: Comparisons Between Alzheimer's Disease Cases and Nondemented Control Subjects," states that "while it is premature to conclude that estrogen replacement therapy is beneficial in this disorder, emerging neurobiological, epidemiological, and clinical evidence raises the possibility that estrogen replacement not only reduces a woman's risk of developing Alzheimer's disease, but the estrogen improves overall cognitive symptoms."

Dr. Howard Fillet, medical director of medicare at New York Life, thinks of Alzheimer's as "osteoporosis of the brain." He explains: "Think of it this way. Estrogen deficiency in the case of osteoporosis leads to fractures thirty years down the road. A woman doesn't really know about her bone loss until finally her hip breaks. Osteoporosis is comparable to the degeneration in the brain. You don't fracture your hip when you're fifty-two, nor do you have dementia. The effect is seen thirty years down the road as more neurons die. It is a chronic degenerative process, and for this reason it makes sense for women to get on estrogen early."

Exciting new research continues to advance our knowledge of estrogen's influence on the body and mind. It seems apparent that once you establish a connection between estrogen and neurotransmitters, it doesn't matter whether you're studying menopause or Alzheimer's. They're separate pieces of the same puzzle. One would think there is little room in this investigation for people blinded by political agendas or medical territorialism. The body is speaking. The question is, will we listen?

# 3

# Menopause and Mental Illness

I was fifty when I had my last period," remembers Rhonda. "Menopause went remarkably well for me. I didn't have hot flashes or any heavy bleeding. I would say I was pretty much free from symptoms and felt fine. Then something started happening to me. I began to feel a strange sort of sadness welling up, a deep melancholy that I couldn't identify or contain. There wasn't any reason for the sadness that I could put my finger on. My life seemed to be going pretty well. I began to notice a definite pattern to this feeling. The mornings would be good. I'd wake up feeling energetic, and would go to work ready for anything. But every day around noon, a wave of unhappiness would wash over me. I began stopping into a local church near my office for solace and reflection. Sometimes it worked, and I'd feel better. But it didn't last; it never did. Nobody could see what was happening to me, because I was too good at hiding it. It kept getting worse, until I thought I was going out of my mind. I finally confided in my internist. I told him what had been happening to me and asked him if he thought it was possible that my feelings were related in any way to my menopause. He assured me that my menopause and my feelings of depression were quite separate issues. They were in no way related. Well, he's an excellent doctor, so I believed him."

*Well, he's an excellent doctor. . . .* I've heard women say this too many times to count. We were raised to have a blind trust in doctors; they inhabited a privileged universe, possessed secrets that were beyond our ability to know or understand. We'd sooner believe a doctor sitting five feet away from us behind a desk than we would the persistent and very real symptoms occurring in our own bodies.

Many women receive inadequate or improper treatment from their physicians and end up feeling helpless or guilty for experiencing entirely treatable physiologically based symptoms. They think it's *their* fault that doctors can't help them! Indeed, when I listen to the stories of women I interviewed, it seems as if doctors were looking everywhere *but* the right place for explanations. And for these particular women, doctors, families, and friends all insisted on seeking solutions from the world of psychiatry.

"It has long been argued that the excess of depression in women is environmental in origin," writes Dr. John W. W. Studd in the *Journal of the North American Menopause Society,*

related to problems with career, family, husband, and feelings of aging. But why is there the sex difference? (Depression is twice as common in women as in men. This excess of depression is seen in population studies, in community studies, hospital admissions, number of suicide attempts and number of prescriptions for anti-depressants.) Is the social, domestic and professional environment really more depressing for a fifty-year-old woman than for a fifty-year-old man? If we fail to acknowledge that a depression in women may have a hormonal basis and as a result avoid asking the appropriate questions about the biology of depression, then we will have failed our patients.

If talking about menopause as a disease state raises the hackles of the politically correct, discussing a link between menopause and depression escalates the controversy tenfold. In spite of the impressive body of research showing a hormonal connection to brain processes, and in spite of the massive clinical evidence that midlife women have statistically high rates of depression, this issue remains an unmentionable in most books about women's health. (If it *is* mentioned, it is only to deny that such a thing as menopausal depression exists.)

It's a touchy subject, even among those who should know better. As of 1989 the *American Journal of Psychiatry* was reporting that "experts now believe menopausal depression is a mythical condition based on unscientific proof." In *American Demographic,* Bonnie Strickland, a psychology professor at the University of Massachusetts, concurs, adding, "Irritation and depression are complaints we hear all the time, whether women are menopausal or not." Even the *Harvard Health Newsletter* has denigrated the notion of menopausal psychiatric illness—albeit with the best of intentions. In an effort to deride early medical texts which depicted all menopausal women as "peevish, irritable, morose, and depressed" and said that many have full-blown insanity with melancholia, paranoia, and maniacal conditions," the editors point out that some modern doctors are merely perpetuating negative images of women with their talk of menopausal madness.

Just last year, Dr. Myrna Lewis, psychiatrist, Mt. Sinai Hospital, New York, addressing a packed audience of women at a conference of the American Menopause Foundation, declared that serious emotional problems at the time of menopause can be traced to three sources: women who have had premenopausal hysterectomies, women with a prior history of depression, and women who may be depressed because of nonrelated events, stresses, and turning points that affect people in their lives. She told the women, "Don't worry about a serious depression. If you have never had one before, you aren't likely to get one as a result of the menopause."

In fact, just the opposite is true. Dr. Lewis's statement is dangerously misleading. Studies show that some women, who are sensitive to the slightest change in hormonal balance, may experience clinical depression in the perimenopause without any previous history of psychological illness.

The critics may have the right motivations. However, the new research on estrogen does not strike the discriminatory tone of ages past, when women were seen as inferior beings under the spell of rampaging hormones at every point in their lives. Indeed, the new data offer a solution to an existing problem that many women have suffered at midlife without hope of relief. In a study of all new clients at a menopause clinic in Edinburgh, Scotland, a clear peak of illness was seen in the perimenopause. Thirty-five percent of patients experienced their first episode of illness during this period. Approximately half of the patients complained that mood changes were their principal disturbance, which they attributed to menopause and for which they wanted help.

In their own studies, Dr. Peter Schmidt and his colleagues at the National Institutes of Health have found no history of past depression in three-quarters of perimenopausal women suffering from major depression. The conclusion is clear. Something occurs during perimenopause that leads to manifestations of clinical depression in a number of women.

"A substantial proportion of perimenopausal women do, in fact, experience a clinically significant depression," says Dr. Schmidt. "Moreover," he continues, "perimenopausal depression may be present in the absence of typical perimenopausal-related symptoms, such as hot flashes." This is important news for physicians. It should also deepen women's understanding of the perimenopausal experience. Estrogen deficiency can be a factor whether or not there are any other recognizable physical symptoms.

To suggest that psychiatric illness in a woman is merely the result of some emotional circumstances in her life, or is a reaction caused by aging, is as cruel as it is wrong. Most women are familiar with the old domino theory—that night sweats and hot flashes cause depression because they interrupt the sleep cycles. No one would argue that sleep interference plays a significant role in compromising one's emotional well-being. But this theory is no longer convincing, since the studies are showing a biochemical basis for depression that is independent of night sweats and hot flashes.

Furthermore, there seems little rationale for viewing clinical depression and psychosis as anything other than organic illness resulting from biological abnormalities. The neurobiological evidence points in that direction. Rockefeller University's Dr.

Bruce McEwen is not surprised that the withdrawal of estrogen for long periods can be a serious problem for some women. "We know a little bit more now about the effects of serotonin, norepinephrine, and dopamine. We know that all of the systems that have major projections through the forebrain seem to have a subtle dependence on estrogen. While estrogen withdrawal is not as complete in some women as in others, based upon body mass and androgen secretions, if you take the estrogens away, not only do synapses disappear in parts of the brain but you are pulling the plug on maintaining some aspects of the function, and possibly the existence, of these major neurotransmitter cells in the brain."

The majority of doctors seem tragically unaware of these findings, glossing over them, failing to understand estrogen's link to psychological illness. Even gynecologists, expected to be on the "front lines" of menopause, often miss the psychological symptoms. After all, OB-GYN specialists did not go into their field expecting to treat this condition, and they may not be equipped, by training or temperament, to care for women with chronic anxiety, depression, irritability, and an inability to cope. They are not always familiar with the medications currently in use, nor are they necessarily prepared to hospitalize someone for menopausally related symptoms. We place most forms of menopausally related illness in their hands, but I have yet to find evidence that it should be there.

Psychiatrists are not likely to make the connection either. They may see women who are experiencing severe psychological symptoms as a result of estrogen deprivation, but on the surface, the symptoms appear to them to be no different from those found in nonmenopausal depressed women.

Physicians must be investigators. They must avoid making casual assumptions and consider all the possibilities. Certainly, if a woman is in the perimenopause, estrogen deficiency should be at the top of the list of potential sources. Furthermore, it is not uncommon in medicine to see similar disorders that have different sources. The symptoms may be the same, but the cause and treatment may be vastly different.

Dr. David Rubinow, of the National Institute of Mental Health, uses the analogy of meningitis to explain this phenomenon. In infants, meningitis is caused by certain bacteria and the treatment is a specific antibiotic. Older people who develop meningitis have the same symptoms as infants, but the disease is contracted from very different bacteria and requires a different antibiotic.

Dr. Edward Klaiber points out that the same holds true for depression in menopause. "The causes of depression before and after menopause may be very different and may require different treatments, although the symptoms are the same. Before menopause, many women respond well to just antidepressants—although our studies show that those premenopausal women who do not respond to antidepressants are often responsive to very high doses of estrogen. After menopause, a combination of estrogen and antidepressants might be appropriate. The bottom line is that physicians should consider estrogen deprivation and inquire about menopausal symptoms."

I confronted my own psychiatrist with questions that had been troubling me. I wanted to know why it had never occurred to him that menopause might be the cause of my illness, and why he hadn't asked for blood tests to check my estrogen levels even earlier than he had. His response was both complimentary and dismaying. "You looked too young," he said. "Besides, we weren't trained that way."

Ironically, the endocrinologist, the one physician specifically trained to comprehend the powerful interplay between estrogen and the brain, seldom has occasion to see menopausal women. Nor are most endocrinologists aware of the vast range of menopausally related symptoms unless they have a specialty in reproductive disease.

"They are not trained to listen to people," says Dr. Michele Harrison, a Boston psychiatrist and family physician. And if there is anything that women with menopause syndrome need, it's to be listened to. "Several years ago, I took a one-week review course in endocrinology at Harvard," she recalls. "The group was almost entirely male. When they started showing slides, I suddenly had a realization. No wonder they think all women are crazy! Endocrinology deals with people whose hormonal levels are clearly off, where people's faces and bodies get funny, where they're oddly shaped—physical manifestations that you can *see*." The endocrinologist, when presented with menopausal symptoms, is dealing with undefined feelings. You can't see feelings. So a woman's report of what she is experiencing may not be manifested in a manner familiar to the endocrinologist.

Hormonal fluctuations during the perimenopause are often overlooked, especially when they are not accompanied by recognizable physical symptoms such as hot flashes. Yet the women I interviewed as I began my research bear witness to the sometimes destructive effects of estrogen deprivation. All these women, though separated dramatically by culture and life experience, are remarkably similar in the problem they were forced to face alone.

In particular, I was struck by the intense shame they felt. Rona experienced terrifying suicidal mood states in her perimenopause. "I was crying a lot," she said, "but since I was still getting my period, my gynecologist thought it was probably PMS. Then the crying and depression got worse, and I started to get anxiety attacks." Rona wondered if she might be menopausal, even though she was still getting her period, so she mentioned it to her gynecologist. He was not sympathetic. "People go through their change of life," he said, "but they don't call me up crying like you do." It was at that point she decided to see a psychiatrist.

"I remember the first time I talked about my depression to friends," Rona said. "I was at work and happened to mention that I was seeing a psychiatrist. 'I am so depressed,' I told them. 'I know something is really wrong.' Two of the women said, 'Oh, for God's sake, we all have periods of depression. We don't run to a doctor for depression.' 'But it's really bad,' I said. They just didn't get it. It made me feel even more isolated.

"It *was* really bad. Even my psychiatrist couldn't help. He gave me Nardil (phenelzine sulfate), and made me promise that I wouldn't do anything stupid. But I was so depressed at that point. I thought to myself, 'I can promise him anything, but I can do what I want to do.' So I made him the promise, but I didn't really mean it. I rode around one night for three hours, thinking about committing suicide. But the next day I was fine. It would come on me like that, and then disappear. I would be as happy as could be and then, for no reason at all, I would get crushingly depressed. I remember one day I was wearing a gold chain, and I suddenly yanked it off my neck and broke it. There was another time when I decided to buy myself a diamond ring.

It was a beautiful estate piece. I was wearing it one day, feeling very happy, when suddenly I just spiraled into a depression. I became so upset that I flung my hand against the wall. I hit it so hard it broke the back of the ring in two. I was devastated.

"Then I was having coffee with a friend one day and telling her about my problems, and she said, 'I think what's happening to you could be a chemical thing. My husband had something years ago where he started acting crazy, and it turned out to be a chemical imbalance.' Her words were magical—and she was right. My psychiatrist finally referred me to an endocrinologist, who discovered my hormonal imbalance. If only I had known where to go from the beginning, I could have spared myself all of the agony I went through. And sometimes I get a shudder and think, I could have *killed* myself!"

## The Great Panic

Panic attacks and depression are often what motivate women to seek professional help. No one ever dies from a panic attack, although the psychological debilitation is so acute that most people feel death is imminent. A panic attack is not just a case of nerves. It is a real physical experience with terrifying symptoms: Your heart races; you feel short of breath; there's a tightening in your chest; your legs are wobbly and uncontrollable. "I thought I was having a heart attack," says the famed country-and-western singer Naomi Judd, who suffered from a series of frightening panic attacks. "It was like I was in mortal danger, struggling to breathe." Unlike women with generalized anxiety, who suffer continuous symptoms, women with panic disorder experience a peak during the attack, which comes on suddenly and usually lasts about twenty minutes.

Since the onset of a panic attack may appear independent of hot flashes, women often miss the hormonal connection. "There are hormonal surges that have the same physiological manifestations as anxiety," observes Dr. Marcia Levy-Warren, a clinical professor of psychology at New York University. "But the women I am most familiar with have not experienced hot flashes, so they haven't considered perimenopause. Some people feel like they're exploding, some people feel like they're suffocating. But the point is that they have real physiological symptoms, with a free-floating sense of impending danger.

Dr. Susan Rako, author of *The Hormone of Desire* (Harmony Books, 1996), has observed that panic attacks may occur during the perimenopause because there is more at work than just a deprivation of estrogen. "There's a hormonal chaos," she says. "Women get spurts of high amounts of estrogen interspersed with low amounts of estrogen. Sometimes the high spikes of estrogen may go on for days at a time. In my observation, those are the periods that seem to be associated with anxiety attacks and the low estrogen with depression and lack of energy."

Studies show that panic and depression are closely linked. Patients with panic disorder and agoraphobia (fear of open spaces) can be depressed; depressed patients can become anxious and phobic, and so on. But they all share symptoms of anxiety that progress from panic attacks to phobias to depressive symptoms.

## The Edge of the Abyss

When depression has spiraled out of control, suicide often looms as the only solution that will end the anxiety and pain. Do hormonal imbalances contribute to the large number of women in their late forties and fifties who take their own lives? According to the statistics gathered by Dr. Alex Crosby, an epidemiologist at the Centers for Disease Control in Atlanta, Georgia, they do. Crosby found that the highest number of female suicides was in the forty- to forty-four-year-old age-group. The second highest number was in the forty-five- to forty-nine-year-old group. The third highest number occurred in the fifty- to fifty-four-year-old age-group, with a dramatic decline in suicide among women between the ages of fifty-four and fifty-nine.

Equally significant are the figures about suicide attempts. In completed suicides, men are three times more successful than women. But when you look at suicide *attempts,* the numbers are reversed. Women attempt suicide three times more often than men.

While biochemical and neuroendocrine breakdowns are particularly prominent in depressed, potentially suicidal women in the perimenopause, all indicators point to serotonin. Studies indicate that there is a correlation between low concentrations of serotonin in the cerebrospinal fluid and suicidal behavior, particularly of an active violent type: hanging, drowning, gas poisoning, several deep cuts. (Drug overdoses by ingestion, single wrist cuts, or combinations of these are considered nonviolent.) Autopsies of suicides of depressed patients as well as autopsies

in patients with other psychiatric conditions also reveal low levels of serotonin. (Lil Traskman, *Arch. Gen. Psychiatry*, 1981.)

Although it is widely assumed that severe depression leads
to suicide, it has been learned that many suicide victims showed
no outward signs of depression before their deaths. When the
fifty-six-year-old wife of New York State senator Frank Padavan
was found hanging in the couple's home, a spokesman reported
that "Mrs. Padavan had been treated for a mild depression. However, there had been nothing in her behavior to indicate that she might do something like this." When a friend's
forty-two-year-old wife was found hanging from her bedroom
ceiling, he agonized over his inability to prevent the tragedy.
"She didn't seem depressed. We had a good life, three terrific
kids, she had a good career. It just happened. She suffered for
as long as I knew her from pretty intense PMS. I have to believe there's some connection there. I just don't understand it
otherwise."

There are three peak times for the onset of moderate to severe
depressive episodes: premenstrually, during the period immediately following childbirth, and in the perimenopausal and
menopausal years. These are all times when the hormones are
out of balance. The most severe reported symptoms seem to
occur in the early perimenopause, in the few years before menstruation ceases altogether or when menopause is surgically induced through a hysterectomy.

The research of Dr. Barbara Sherwin, at McGill University,
supports these findings. "One of the studies we undertook used
perimenopausal women about to have total hysterectomies for

reasons other than benign disease. All of the women were otherwise healthy. There was no history of psychiatric illness, no history of psychotropic drug use, and they were all in stable personal relationships.

"After their surgery," she said, "some of the women were given hormone replacement therapy and some were given a placebo. All of the women receiving hormone replacement showed markedly better overall moods than those women receiving the placebo medication. And in the fourth month of treatment, when the hormone was withdrawn altogether, the women who had been receiving it all along showed clear evidence of depression. The message of the study was crystal clear."

## It's All in the Hormones

When women present themselves to doctors reporting depression, panic attacks, or suicidal impulses, why do they have so much trouble getting correctly diagnosed? Obviously, because everyone around them, including the doctors, thinks they are mentally ill—and so do the women themselves. Why would clinically depressed women, much less psychotic or suicidal women, seek relief in a gynecologist's office or at a menopause clinic? They would probably be referred to a psychiatrist or psychiatric hospital for treatment. Many years ago, when the Swiss physician V. S. Burgi decided to study chronic postpartum illness, he found plenty of subjects in the back wards of psychiatric hospitals. Since it is well documented that perimenopausal hormonal changes can evoke symptoms similar to postpartum psychiatric illness, we may discover to our horror that clinically depressed and psychotic menopausal women can be found not only in psychiatrists' offices but locked up in the psychiatric units of our own community hospitals.

That is why the research by Dr. Klaiber and his colleagues at Worcester State Hospital is unique and so critically important. The women in their study were already considered mentally ill. They would never turn up at a gynecologist's office or a clinic. The only logical way to identify this patient population was through psychiatric channels.

"Gynecologists almost never see the seriously ill psychiatric patient," Dr. Klaiber observes. "Those are seen by psychiatrists who rarely recognize the hormonal component. It requires a cross-disciplinary effort by various medical specialists to approach this problem, and, as we know all too well, cross-disciplinary efforts are often difficult to arrange, particularly between specialists who don't often communicate with one another, such as the psychiatrist and the gynecologist."

It's easy to see how insidious the problem becomes. The sad irony for the woman suffering from a hormonally based psychosis is that the doctor she will most likely turn to may be the last person who is really able to help her.

Another reason many women have trouble getting help is that their symptoms just don't seem serious enough—at least in the beginning. Maybe they're feeling a little down, or having trouble concentrating, or feeling tired. How easily these women's symptoms are dismissed as "just signs of aging."

But some of the symptoms, such as the sudden forgetfulness that can occur during menopause, are frightening. My friend Ann, a fellow high school English teacher, told me about her own experience. "I was in the middle of a class lesson on syntax, and suddenly the word just slipped out of my brain or something! I couldn't believe it. How many years have I been doing this? 'Oh my Lord,' I thought to myself, 'the end must be near. It must be the first sign of Alzheimer's disease.' I didn't panic at all. I just crumbled."

"There are thousands of menopausal women who aren't feeling quite well," Dr. Klaiber reports. "They aren't sleeping well, their moods are erratic, they're having difficulty with their cognitive skills. This isn't unusual. A friend of mine was telling me just the other day that his wife is suddenly having a problem with grocery shopping. She can't seem to make up her mind what brand of an item to get and so is spending increasing amounts of time at the supermarket. I recognized this problem immediately. The studies we're currently working on clearly reveal that women on estrogen make decisions faster, are more accurate, and are more confident overall. So many of the women in my study have started out by saying, 'There's nothing wrong with my mind.' Then, after they've been on estrogen for a few months, they come back and say, 'You know, Dr. Klaiber, I think there was something wrong with my mind before.' It never fails, and, frankly, I'm pleased to do anything I can to restore a sense of well-being to women whose lives have virtually been shattered by unrecognized endocrine problems. Hormone replacement therapy has acted like a miracle cure for many women who otherwise would have spent their lives locked away in psychiatric units and permanently encased in a haze of psychotropic medications."

## The Prozac Problem

It's clear that women's efforts to find help are complicated by the fact that we live in the quick-fix "Prozac era." Since Dr. Peter Kramer wrote the best-seller *Listening to Prozac* in 1992, Prozac and other mood enhancers or antidepressants have become ubiquitous. Today millions of people take antidepressants as casually as they take vitamins.

Not surprisingly, many of the women I have interviewed reported having Prozac or Zoloft prescribed for their depression, moodiness, panic attacks, and anxiety. In some cases they found minor temporary relief. But Prozac did not reverse their primary symptoms, nor did it address any of the physical problems that often accompanied them. Carla's experience was typical.

Carla's sense of complete exhaustion and inappropriate outbursts of anger alerted her to the onset of her perimenopause. Whenever her menstrual cycle began, she would literally take to her bed. "I was wiped out," she explains. "I couldn't believe it. I'd never had any problems with my period or anything else. I wasn't anemic. I'd always been a good sleeper—and then this. But that wasn't even the worst of it. Suddenly I began to feel that my basic personality, my temperament, was undergoing some kind of terrible change. I never knew how I'd react to things, and there were incidents that were just scary. I'd start arguing with my perfectly nice sister-in-law about some obscure piece of family trivia and end up sobbing in the bathroom. Or I'd disagree with someone during a meeting at work and walk out. None of this was *me*. I couldn't figure out what was going on, so I finally went to see my internist. He didn't take any blood tests or ask me questions about my cycles, or even address my physical symptoms. Within minutes of my walking into his office, I was on my way out again with a prescription for Prozac. Of course, I was ready to try anything, and I had heard about the supposed miracle properties of this drug. I took it religiously for two months, and *nothing* changed."

Carla continued to have problems for many months. She went from doctor to doctor, until one finally suggested that her symptoms might be hormonally related. Indeed they were. Blood tests showed that Carla was severely estrogen deprived. With appropriate treatment, Carla's problems quickly came under control. She now looks back on that period as a time of unnecessary torment, and she is angry with the internist who so quickly prescribed Prozac. "I realize now that he either didn't believe any of my physical symptoms were real or he just wasn't listening to me. In fact, I'm sure that he thought I was having some sort of an emotional breakdown."

If doctors were "listening to estrogen as closely as they were listening to Prozac, they might see the distinction between the two drugs. Both act on serotonin, the primary neurotransmitter that controls moods. *But if you have an estrogen deficiency, Prozac will not be effective.* Estrogen deficiency causes the receptors for serotonin to deteriorate. So even though Prozac increases a woman's level of serotonin, she has no receptor for Prozac to work on. Without estrogen, Prozac is ineffective. In fact, only when women who had failed to respond to at least two antidepressants were treated with estrogen in combination with an antidepressant did their depressive symptoms diminish.

The receptors had to be stimulated by estrogen in order to work properly. This is the key issue surrounding the use of Prozac and other antidepressants to treat psychiatric disorders in estrogen-deficient menopausal women.

There is another major difference between the actions of Prozac and estrogen. Prozac inhibits serotonin reuptake—meaning that it prevents serotonin from being absorbed back into its original nerve endings, thus strengthening its concentration at the synapses. But estrogen actually *controls* the enzyme (tryptophane hydroxylase, or TPH) that *makes* serotonin. This finding is the result of a study just completed at the Oregon Regional Primate Research Center. Dr. Cynthia Bethea, one of the authors of the study, explains the excitement: "It provides, for the first time, evidence of a biological influence for mood disorders related to reproductive function in women at a molecular level. It's a major breakthrough. The data provided by these studies are particularly relevant to women because of the use of a nonhuman primate, the rhesus monkey, which has a reproductive cycle and a serotonin network in the brain that closely resembles that of humans."

Other studies confirm the influence of estrogen on serotonin production. In fact, researchers have found that low TPH is associated with severe maternity blues, suggesting that estrogen deficiency is the precipitating factor. Severe maternity blues might be the model not only for early postpartum psychotic depression but for PMS, menopausal psychiatric illness, and even Alzheimer's disease.

Many of the women who seek medical intervention for their psychiatric symptoms should first be thoroughly examined and

tested by a clinician who will seek signs of a hormonal imbalance. If more women began treatment with a prescription for
estrogen rather than one for antidepressant or antipsychotic
drugs, there would be clear and overwhelming evidence that for
most menopausal women, mood brighteners like Prozac are beside the point. Dr. Kramer suggests in *Listening to Prozac* that
both Prozac and estrogen are mood brighteners in that they en-
hance or transform normal functioning. But the issues are not
parallel. For perimenopausal women with psychiatric illness, the
goal is to restore normal functioning. These women, who have
lost all sense of their former selves, would happily settle for
being "normal" again. Estrogen is not a mood brightener; it is
a mood restorer that is responding to a depletion state.

# 4

## *Marcia:*
## Living an Alternate Reality

I lay stretched out on my bed, limp and exhausted, as if I had been drugged with a powerful narcotic. The late summer sun streaked in through the curtains of my bedroom. This was once my favorite time of the year—the mellow days at the end of summer in Stockbridge. Now I barely noticed the time of year or the world around me. During the past three days I had been immersed in an alternate reality. I had been allowed very little food or rest. With each passing day, the commands grew harsher and more humiliating. The biblical passage I had memorized was a precursor to a nightmare period during which I was repeatedly forced to perform degrading rituals of purification and cleansing, after which I would collapse in a heap. I'd barely doze off before I was pulled awake again. I was vaguely aware that school was to begin the following day, and I needed to get back to Fort Lee, New Jersey, and make preparations. But I couldn't will myself to move.

From what seemed millions of miles away, I heard the phone begin to ring. It was the first time since the voices had taken control of me that an exterior reality had intruded. I had long since given myself over in numbed submission, but the sound of the ringing phone cut into my delusional world, wrenching me back.

I recall standing in the kitchen with a sheet draped around me. I must have pulled it off the bed before racing up the circular staircase from the bedroom to answer the phone. I also had the Ouija board with me.

It was my daughter-in-law, Beth, calling to tell me that she and Douglas had arrived in Cleveland and settled into their new apartment. I struggled desperately to keep our conversation normal, but I was having trouble responding like myself. Our call was being monitored by the powers that now controlled me. I began shaking involuntarily. I was afraid that I wouldn't be able to keep my new world a secret. I had to be sure that no one suspected anything.

When I hung up the telephone, I was convinced that I had pulled it off. Only later would I learn that what I thought had been a normal conversation with my daughter-in-law was the first of several alarming exchanges with those who were closest to me. Still, it had required my total concentration to keep from cutting the phone call short. I was obsessed with the need to get back to the board. And now there was an even more compelling reason. I needed permission from it to return to New Jersey. I reached across the kitchen counter for the Ouija board and pulled it toward me, placing my hand on the pointer. Even as the pointer whipped around the board, I knew I didn't feel strong enough to negotiate my request to return home, and I was highly agitated. Then I heard the voice of God say,

MARCIA, YOU MAY RETURN TO NEW JERSEY. BUT KEEP THE OUIJA BOARD BESIDE YOU. WE WILL CONTINUE OUR WORK TOGETHER WHEN YOU ARRIVE HOME.

Afraid that He might change His mind, I raced downstairs, and, leaving the bed in crumpled disarray and a bathroom littered with plastic bottles, Vaseline jars askew, towels, and tissues strewn across the floor, I grabbed my suitcase out of the closet, gathered my things, and left Stockbridge for my apartment in Fort Lee. The Ouija board sat next to me in the car all the way home.

It would be another week before the voices would disappear. Even though my inner world was coexisting with the real world, there was still a separation between them that I understood. Once I was at home in New Jersey, I was aware of my functional public life, but it was my inner world that made me feel intensely alive. It had a symmetry and integrity that made absolute sense to me, even though I knew no one else could or would understand it. So it had to be kept secret. (Besides, I knew it would be dangerous for me if it were revealed without God's permission.) But it was a strenuous effort, for part of me was no longer anchored to everyday things. I was tormented by my need to monitor my behavior so I wouldn't give myself away.

In the quiet early morning of my first day back, stretched across my bed, I was like a swimmer carried away from shore in an undertow, stranded in the powerful pull of my inner life. I buried myself deeper under my comforter. I wanted to crawl back into myself to a place where no one could find me, even though I knew my first class of the school year was only hours away. School felt like an intrusion on my *real* life. I hated the thought of dealing with the other reality. As I prepared to leave the sanctuary of my apartment, I felt as if part of me were about to be amputated.

I have no way to explain what it was that kept me glued to life in the coming days. I came as close as anyone could to psychological disintegration, yet I kept on going. I was like a bionic machine whose activating switch was stuck in overdrive. I was capable of tremendous endurance, and I was never tired. Even in a raging psychotic state, I managed to drive from Fort Lee to Long Island every morning, leaving my apartment at 6:45 to teach a full day. When I wasn't teaching, time seemed to suspend itself and the days would become endless. Even when I collapsed into sleep, in the early hours before dawn, I was always up just a few hours later. Sleep deprivation was a fundamental part of my illness, and I would later learn that the rhythm of sleep is commonly disrupted by estrogen deprivation.

The first day of school was a test of will, but the drive to Long Island calmed me somewhat. The trip across the George Washington and Throgs Neck Bridges to the Cross Island Parkway was so familiar to me that it was as if my car were moving on automatic pilot. Lulled by the lilting motion of the car as it slipped around each bend in the road, I was surprised when suddenly I found myself in full view of the high school. Then it hit me: I was going to walk in there and have to deal with people for the first time. People who knew me. Would they be able to see any difference in me? I became anxious and distracted. I swung my car into the parking lot adjacent to the school and pulled into my assigned space. With my hands trembling, I reached for the Ouija board. I was in desperate need of reassurance, but no sooner had I touched the board than I noticed that cars had pulled in on either side of me. Frantic at the thought of being exposed, I hurriedly covered the board with a sweater, making certain no part of it was visible. Then I gathered up my things, trying to be inconspicuous, and headed toward the entrance to the school, taking long, deep breaths to calm my nerves. As ill as I was, I was aware that my public image demanded certain conventions. I knew that I could never lose control. It would require every ounce of energy to do that. I was undertaking a precarious balancing act. Irrational forces were dominating my life, subverting me to their demands. At any moment I was in danger of disengaging totally. I was living a desperate and hazardous existence.

It never occurred to me that the degree to which I worried about being exposed far exceeded the likelihood of that happening. The range of what is considered normal behavior is so open to interpretation that what clinicians label madness others view as merely eccentric—or, to draw a parallel from Hannah Arendt, perhaps there is a banality in madness as well as in evil that masks it from the common eye. So it is unremarkable how often in our ordinary lives human suffering goes undetected.

The irony of my situation was both pitiful and tragic. I had a chance to get help. I was surrounded by students, colleagues, and friends; yet I felt imprisoned in my mind, unable to reach out for that help. In fact, I felt terribly threatened by my friends. I had created a psychic boundary that others could not penetrate. It was my invisible "line in the sand," across which everyone I encountered was a potential enemy, capable of discovering my secret, threatening to expose me.

Had I been less experienced in teaching, I might have given myself away. But fifteen years in the classroom had enabled me to maneuver easily through my routine, and there was nothing to indicate that I was acting in any way out of the ordinary.

But if no one noticed anything unusual about *me,* I was viewing *them* through a warped screen. Everyone and everything around me was infused with an unreal quality. I felt myself gradually becoming distanced from reality, as if the visible world was fading before my eyes. It required a strenuous effort for me to stay connected.

In fact, in spite of the ease with which I handled my first class, by late morning the delusions had deepened. Midway through my second class, God's voice suddenly manifested itself in my head. It was as if someone cut in on a party line; suddenly I was trying to carry on two conversations at once. I thought that God was monitoring my teaching! I grew anxious, afraid that He would be displeased. I was distracted, straining to hear some word in my mind that would signal His approval. But the sign I received was not the one I had anticipated.

As I continued to explain a point to my class, an eruption occurred inside me. Deep within my body I felt a familiar undulating motion, then strong, rapid uterine contractions that signaled God's presence and were not in my own power. I was filled with longing, feelings that seemed to arise from my sense of helplessness, and though there was as yet no outward sign of the war raging in my mind, my situation was precarious. God was gaining ascendancy, and my controls were deteriorating. The extreme pressure of school was exacerbating my delusion. In a matter of hours, my behavior would be completely bizarre.

In the interval between classes I immediately withdrew to the English center. I settled myself at a large mahogany desk at one end of the room, feeling relief from the strain of trying to concentrate all my energy on teaching, answering questions, and engaging in ordinary conversation. As I sat there, I began to feel a deep need to consult the Ouija board, which I had left locked in my car. I reached into my bag for my car keys and discovered they were missing.

I rummaged through my purse, fingering my way around familiar objects heaped together, poking into pockets in corners of the lining, and becoming increasingly agitated. I turned my bag over on the table, spilling out its contents, but there was still no sign of the keys. So I shoved everything back, flung my bag over my shoulder, and hurried out of the room in a mad race to retrace my steps, darting in and out of places where I thought I might have dropped the keys, finally stopping at the main office to see whether anyone had turned them in. But no one had—or so I thought. I later learned that the assistant principal had found them, tossed them into a drawer, and promptly forgot about them.

I was increasingly on edge as I walked back to the English center. I wondered whether I had dropped my keys in the driveway next to the car, and then the thought occurred to me that I might have left them in the ignition. I was flustered and anxious, but I had only a few minutes until my last class of the day, so I sat back down at my desk.

Suddenly I felt a rush of excitement. I thought my eyes were deceiving me at first, but from where I sat there was no mistaking it. I could make out the familiar black and white design of a Ouija board box set on top of a filing cabinet across from where I was sitting. I was stunned by the irony of its appearance in the room. But I was also so giddy and pleased with the thought that the English center conferred on the Ouija board a certain legitimacy, a kind of academic seal of approval. I was amazed and convinced that the appearance of the Ouija board was no accident. I became obsessed with the idea that seemingly ordinary circumstances were being manipulated by God, that they were tests of my faith and obedience.

I was self-conscious about my discovery, and since I noticed that there were other teachers in the room, I knew I had to find a way to get access to the board without giving myself away. I decided to confront the matter head-on. As I strode across the room and pulled the box off the cabinet, I casually exclaimed to no one in particular, "What on earth is this doing here?" (It would be some months before I learned that the Ouija board had been purchased years earlier as an amusing distraction for what was otherwise a serious unit on literature and the supernatural.)

Feigning curiosity that such a bizarre item would have found its way into the English center, I jauntily carried it to where I was sitting and lifted the board out of the box. Then I asked offhandedly, "What do you imagine this thing is all about?" Whoever was present in the room was indifferent to my questions There were quizzical looks and some shrugs of the shoulders, but no one expressed any serious interest. So I eagerly pulled the Ouija onto my lap and began to work the board. As soon as I did, the pointer began to sweep around the letters in convoluted movement. The message surprised me. It said to take the Ouija board into the girls' bathroom and work it in the privacy of one of the stalls.

I was high-spirited as I gathered up my things and hastened across the hall to the girls' bathroom. I headed for one of the cubicles at the far end of the room, slipped inside, and fastened the lock. Then I eased myself down on the edge of the toilet seat lid and placed the Ouija board across my knees. The moment my hand touched the pointer, my arm surged forward and began to whip around the board. I could feel my excitement mount as the words started to form under the clear plastic eye, yet the instructions were bizarre.

I was told that I would find my keys under one of the cars in the driveway, adjacent to the school. At the end of the school day, I was to search carefully under each one—about eighty cars—and I would find my keys. While I somehow sensed that this was God's way of demonstrating His power to materialize objects at will, I also felt as if the circumstances surrounding my keys were another test of my obedience. But no matter how God made his presence known to me, my spirit soared. I felt as if I were billowing into space.

I struggled through my final class, operating on some other frequency. Even hours later, as I walked the length of the driveway, the steady stream of teachers who were heading for their cars had little effect on my mood. It never occurred to me to wonder if anyone thought my behavior was out of the ordinary. Other people were no longer a source of embarrassment for me;

they were an inconvenience I could not ignore. Occasionally, when someone caught my attention, I reminded myself to smile, but otherwise I was detached and preoccupied.

I was gradually becoming aware of the number of cars that had already left the school, and I was experiencing mounting tension in the expectation of finding my keys, when suddenly, in the midst of examining the pavement under one of the few remaining cars, I spun upright. At the barest threshold of awareness, I could hear a faint whisper in my head repeating the word TREES over and over. I stood motionless, straining to hear if there were something more. That's when I heard the message:

THE TREES, MARCIA.

YOUR KEYS ARE UNDER A TREE.

SEE IF YOU CAN IDENTIFY WHICH ONE IT IS.

I looked around in all directions, staking out the school grounds. Across the parking lot, toward the entrance to the school, there were elm trees that scaled the height of the two-story building. Their thick branches, stretching across the width of the school, created a fanciful lattice effect. *Those must be the trees,* I thought, hurrying past some students who were heading in the opposite direction. Then, as if to achieve an attitude of nonchalance, I slipped out of my shoes and, gathering them up in my hand, walked barefoot across the front law of the school, buoyed with the promise of at last recovering my keys. It was a bizarre ceremony as I threaded my way from tree to tree, kneeling at the base of each one, separating the tufts of grass, searching the ground with my fingers. The day was very warm for September, more like an August afternoon that had been put aside and trotted out unexpectedly for a final backward glance toward summer, and its effect on me was enervating. I could feel a pounding at my temples, and perspiration rolled down from my forehead and trickled into the corners of my eyes, causing them to blur. I became irritated, frustrated by my inability to see. The low humming in my ears continued, and at first it masked the voice that suddenly resounded in my head as if it had surfaced from some hollowed-out chamber.

I stood up straight, gripped by fear.

GO TO YOUR CAR, MARCIA. THE GAME IS OVER.

I swung around, robotlike, and walked some distance to where my car was parked, angled toward a chain-link fence, peculiarly isolated. I felt as if I were being carried in the throes of something that filled me with a sense of fatality, and I had barely the presence of mind to put on my shoes before stepping into the driveway. I was being prodded, pushed along by some inexorable force. But it was the cryptic quality of His words that filled me with dread, their stark simplicity.

GET INTO YOUR CAR, MARCIA, AND LOCK THE DOOR.

I pulled the door handle and was surprised to find that the car was unlocked. I got in, slammed the door shut, and locked it. I pushed aside the sweater covering the Ouija board and seized the pointer. It felt as if an unseen hand were pulling my arm toward the board, and I sensed suddenly that I was in the presence of a malignant force. But there was no way I could have prepared for His message:

PUT BACK THE SEAT, MARCIA, NOW YOU ARE GOING TO DIE.

My mind was arrested, stunned by His words. I felt the total control He had over me, and I lay back in the car. Bracing my feet against the floor where it curved behind the pedals, I experienced for the first time a vague sense of my own destruction. Time seemed to suspend itself, and a stillness crept over me. I could feel my body begin to shut down.

The sun beat through the airtight windows, and I lay motionless in the silence. In that interval, I recall visualizing the faces of my colleagues, noses flattened against my car window, straining to get a glimpse of my lifeless body limp against the seat.

Then, God's voice abruptly thundered through my mind, and I heard His solemn pronouncement:

YOU CAN SIT UP, MARCIA, I HAVE DECIDED TO LET YOU LIVE. DO WHATEVER YOU NEED TO DO. WE WILL GO TO WORK WHEN YOU GET HOME.

There is no way to communicate what it's like to be given such a reprieve, to be recalled to life. I was wildly excited. But I still lay there for some time without moving, concentrating on my breathing. Finally, I pulled the lever to raise my seat to a sitting position and slowly shifted my body upright. But I could sense that something was wrong; then I realized that I couldn't move my legs. I tried, but they remained frozen in place. My knees were clamped shut, like jaws clenched together. Then I realized that, in an effort to gain control, to alleviate my terror, I had transferred my fear to my legs. I had pushed my full weight against them, keeping the tension at its most penetrating intensity the entire time I lay outstretched.

I concentrated on relaxing, gently flexing my knees, and eased them to a sitting position. Then I pulled on the door handle and in one accelerated sweep of motion pushed it open and staggered out of the car. My legs began to buckle under me, and I leaned against the fender for support.

In the time I had imprisoned myself in the car, the sun pouring through the windows, I had become drenched in perspiration. As I leaned against the car, feeling my clothes wet and heavy against my body, I was suddenly distracted by a splash of color visible in the distance. I could make out a dress, a swirl of flaming orange, which I immediately recognized as belonging to a cheerleader. She seemed to me like a vision, her blond hair falling loose over her shoulders, the blue and orange pom-poms on her sneakers bouncing up and down as she half-skipped across the sidewalk in the direction of the school. I was overcome with a desire to run toward her and throw my arms around her. I anticipated the thrill of connecting to something alive, something real—wrenched as I was from a dark and suffocating place. This intense need for physical contact became a dominant part of my waking life and remained with me over the next several weeks.

Powerful unconscious forces had somehow transformed the way I viewed the world around me. Now when I walked along the street, I would watch the people moving past me, going about the routine of their lives, and it was as if filaments of gauze, ever so transparent, had fallen between us. I felt dead within my space, and I wanted only to reach out and grab the people close to me. I needed to absorb their aliveness.

Today, as my mind reaches back to that dark period, I am suddenly aware that fear has vanished altogether, and in its place I am filled with a terrible sadness. I can only shake my head, bewildered by how I could have allowed myself to endure such needless suffering. Indeed, I can barely comprehend the waste of such a magnificent outpouring of energy. There is no experience—*none*—in the range of human existence that can

rival the irony of a breakdown. When else would a person believe herself to be a victim while all she is going through is simply her own invention? When else would a person plan terrible
ways of punishing herself, and in desperate straits, given enough
time, devise the means to become her own executioner?

# 5

# The Female Continuum

To understand more about what was happening to me, and what has happened to countless other women, let's step back for a moment and follow the hormonal trail. It is an unbroken yet mazelike passage, stretching from menarche to menopause, through stages and cycles that seem distinct but are actually part of a single continuum. Since hormonal activity is always a vital presence, it is realistic to conclude that hormonal imbalances can set off psychoses at every point along the trail. We must begin looking at conditions such as severe PMS and postpartum psychosis as hormonally driven.

In her stirring book, *The Adolescent Journey*, Dr. Marcia Levy-Warren observes that in many ways midlife is a "recapitulation of adolescence . . . by its nature, a time when limitations, symbolic deaths, and explosiveness are prominent developmental issues." Dr. Levy-Warren concludes that menopausal women are dealing with the flip side of the hormonal coin—the end of their childbearing years. There is bound to be some emotional fallout, as all life passages strike primordial chords. But the biological picture is more complex than that. The hormonal impact, at every stage, is not just related to childbearing.

It is, however, related to cyclical patterns. The connection between estrogen deprivation in menopause and its effect on mood and behavior can be traced to the *timing* of the symptoms. The hormonal changes in women who have PMS, which has been classified as a psychiatric illness, and the biochemical changes responsible for postpartum depression are cyclical in nature. Timing speaks even more powerfully than the symptoms themselves. Premenstrual syndrome occurs in the late phase of the menstrual cycle, when the ovaries are most actively producing female hormones. Postpartum depression usually occurs within the six months following delivery, with the loss of the placenta, the body's source of estrogen. Menopausal depression occurs when the ovaries cease producing estrogen. Could there be any clearer examples of cause and effect?

"The time that estrogen reaches its lowest point premenstrually, 35 percent of women experience moderate physical and psychological symptoms of depression and 3 percent experience severe incapacitating symptoms," reports Dr. Barbara Sherwin. "Following the one-hundred-fold decrease in circulating estrogen and progesterone levels which occurs after childbirth, 50 to 70 percent of women experience a mild, transient mood disorder on the third to tenth postpartum day, 10 to 15 percent of women experience a major depressive disorder within the first three postpartum months, and .1 to .2 percent of women experience a postpartum psychosis. And, of course, the third reproductive event that is characterized by a fairly drastic decrease in circulating estrogen levels, is the menopause."

If we could graph the brain, charting the shifts that occur in each of the major reproductive transitions in women's lives, we would be able to measure, precisely, the changes in their hormone levels. What would surely emerge would be an overarching pattern, a direct pathway from one female transition to another, showing the role that estrogen plays in triggering psychiatric illness in predisposed women, premenstrually, postpartum, perimenopausally, postmenopausally, in surgical menopause, and in Alzheimer's disease. If we could chart these shifts, it would be heartening to contemplate the advances that could be made. Women who are struggling through periods of emotional devastation that are hormonally triggered could be spared the disruption and pain that they have needlessly endured.

## The Estrogen-Progesterone Cycle

A typical menstrual cycle occurs over twenty-eight days, with a hormonal ebb and flow. The first five days are the menstrual period, when the endometrium—the lining of the uterus—is shed. During menstruation, the female hormones, estrogen and progesterone, are at their lowest levels. During the sixth through the eleventh days, the estrogen levels continue to rise, surging around the twelfth day and then beginning to decline again. Within approximately thirty-six hours of the estrogen surge—

about the fourteenth day—ovulation occurs. This fourteen-day period is referred to as the *follicular* phase.

The last fourteen days of the cycle are known as the *luteal* phase. During this period estrogen levels drop while progesterone levels rise. Progesterone is the hormone that prepares the uterine lining for pregnancy, in the event that an egg has been fertilized. If no fertilization occurs, it is this lining that is sloughed off during the menstrual period.

Premenstrual symptoms, ranging from mild to severe, occur during the luteal phase, when progesterone is high and estrogen is low. These symptoms may include erratic moods and depression. The impairment of serotonin function because of lowered estrogen levels is responsible for depressive illness in the perimenopause and postpartum, and a growing body of evidence indicates that serotonin function is also impaired on a cyclical basis in premenstrual syndrome.

However, there are differences of opinion about how to treat cyclical depressive illness. Many doctors believe that PMS-related depression should be treated with progesterone. At first blush, this may appear to make no sense, since the progesterone levels are already high, and it is the estrogen levels that are depleted. But there seems to be a threshold of tolerance beyond which progesterone has a completely different pharmacologic effect on the brain.

According to Dr. Elizabeth Vliet, in high doses progesterone has been found to be about eight times more potent as an anti-anxiety and sedative agent than the most potent barbiturate known today, methohexital. Studies have also found it more potent than Klonopin, a high-potency drug used for epilepsy and panic disorder. At high levels it actually acts very much like anti-anxiety medications, such as Xanax or Valium.

Not all doctors agree that high doses of progesterone can help decrease anxiety in some women with severe PMS. In fact, there is a clear divide in the medical community over the efficacy of progesterone as a prophylactic. Some physicians feel that the level of thinking on this matter relegates it to medical antiquity. "If progesterone has any role in PMS," Dr. John Studd writes in "Estrogens and Depression in Women," "it is one of causation. Treating PMS with progesterone is like bleeding for anemia."

Dr. Andrew Herzog, a neurologist at Beth Israel Hospital in Boston, emphasizes the potential danger for some women in any reproductive transition when their balance of estrogen and progesterone is compromised. He was one of the pioneers in the 1970s who recognized the effects of hormonal imbalance on women prone to epileptic seizures. Women kept saying that their seizures varied with their menstrual cycle. They were right. Dr. Herzog explains that for some women, long intervals of un-opposed estrogen can trigger seizures. Women who are prone to seizures or anxiety disorders need to have their estrogen balanced with progesterone.

We do not have a thorough understanding of the myriad hormonal pathways to the brain. Scientists have yet to perfect their understanding of the specific effects of estrogen and progesterone, either alone or in combination. But those who have been studying these pathways are certain of one thing: The effect of hormonal imbalance is powerful, and it can be devastating to the women whose reactions to the unique hormonal fluctuations of their bodies are not understood.

Let's examine some of the true experiences that so many young girls and adult women go through—and have gone through for years.

## The First Stage: Adolescence

We often refer to "exploding hormones" when we talk about what causes teenage behavioral problems. We even joke about it. But until recently no one thought to study the cyclical nature of physical and emotional symptoms in teenage girls.

Dr. I. Ronald Shenker, professor of pediatrics at Albert Einstein College of Medicine and chief of Adolescent Medicine at Long Island Jewish Hospital, thinks that's a shame. Dr. Shenker has found that too often girls who exhibit behavioral problems are being misidentified as emotionally disturbed when the source of the problem is hormonal. These girls need their cycles regulated, not their lives upended.

"We see kids who are depressed and who have conduct disorders and other manifestations that are not explicable at our current state of knowledge on physical changes and physical alterations," Dr. Shenker explains. "I am convinced that the more we look, the more we're going to find that the behavior is organically induced. We should study the organic and the psychological together, rather than focusing on one or the other."

It seems maddeningly simple, yet this solution seems to elude both medical doctors and psychiatrists. In the rare cases when a doctor is sensitive to the possibility of a hormonal connection, the results are gratifying. Years before my own breakdown, I ex-

perienced this directly with my student Sheila. From the very beginning of the school year, Sheila, age fifteen, had seemed unusually sullen and withdrawn. She appeared distracted, troubled
about something. I was concerned, because this just wasn't like
her. She had always been a serious student, and I was alarmed
when she started slipping behind. When Sheila missed a test and
came to see me about arranging a makeup, I expressed my concern. She shyly confided that her mother had taken her to the
doctor for some blood work. They were trying to find out if
there was a hormonal reason for her sudden problems. I was in-
trigued; it hadn't occurred to me to think of hormones. A few
days later Sheila told me that a hormonal imbalance was indeed
discovered, and she'd been placed on estrogen replacement therapy. At fifteen! I had never heard of such a thing, and I was fas-
cinated by the story Sheila and her mother told me many months
after she was back to normal.

Sheila described her struggle to cope with the sudden and terrifying changes that had started during the summer—changes
that were both powerful and inexplicable. "I got real down at
the beginning of last summer, right after school let out," she told
me. "That was also right after the last time I got my period. I
started having bad moods, good moods—I'd be really happy,
suddenly I'd get really mad, start crying and stuff. I couldn't
sleep that well, so I was sort of cranky. But what flipped me out
the most was . . . maybe I shouldn't say. I was freaked. I mean,
I suddenly had hair growing on my lip! It was disgusting!"

By the time the school year started, Sheila was feeling worse
than ever. "I couldn't think. I couldn't concentrate," she said. "I

didn't care how I looked, I didn't care what I wore. I didn't want to hang out with anybody. I would just start crying all the time. It was really bad."

Meanwhile, her mother was noticing a lot of disturbing changes in her daughter. "Sheila was this sweet, gorgeous, energetic girl, and all of a sudden she was exhausted all the time, waking up tired every day," she recalled. "She was very moody. She's never been difficult, but all of sudden, she was unhappy, sad, jumpy. I thought maybe she had Lyme disease. I didn't know."

Then Sheila's mother noticed that her daughter seemed to be gaining weight, but it wasn't a normal weight gain. "She was getting bigger, muscular, like an athlete. And she wasn't working out or anything. Also, I saw that she was suddenly getting very hairy all over her body. Her upper lip, chin, and stomach. And her periods were irregular, for the first time. Sheila had started menstruating when she was eleven, and she'd never had a problem before. That's when I started to think it might be a female thing."

Sheila's mother finally called their gynecologist, who immediately did blood work and determined that she was estrogen deficient. The doctor placed Sheila on a low-dosage birth control pill to counter the hormonal imbalance and to help regulate her periods.

It took a couple of weeks, but it worked. "I started to feel *normal,*" Sheila said with relief. "I'd been miserable for so long! I forgot how much happier I could feel. I started sleeping better, I stopped feeling so bummed, and I stopped feeling so jumpy I could die. My body started looking like *me* again—no more of that disgusting hair!"

Sheila's experience reveals with bracing clarity the potentially devastating effects of destabilized hormone levels on an adolescent girl. If she is predisposed to psychiatric illness, the result can be catastrophic. While family history may offer clues, there is no definitive means to identify the hypersensitive. These hormonal shifts may account for a girl's "acting out," her inability to concentrate in class, falling grades, and family conflicts. School records which monitor absenteeism may reveal a cyclical pattern relevant to a hormonal problem. In any case, counselors, teachers, and parents should be alerted to the possibility of some underlying endocrine factor.

Sheila's experience confirms that junior high and high schools may be the best laboratories in which to study the effects of hormonal imbalances on adolescent girls. There are probably many teenage girls suffering from such ailments as sleep disturbances, anxiety attacks, and mood swings. Their symptoms may run the gamut from mild to severe depression and may be dismissed simply as "an adolescent thing," when the real problem is a severe hormonal imbalance.

More alarming still is that psychiatric illness in adolescent girls is generally not recognized as a hormonally related condition. In fact, one of the potential hazards for women who experience a hormonally induced psychotic episode during adolescence and later is that they may present constellations of symptoms that resemble those of a mental illness. The resulting treatment with the present daunting array of antipsychotic medications may prove that maxim "Sometimes the cure is worse than the disease."

One case reported to the *British Journal of Psychiatry* involved a fourteen-year-old girl who manifested all the features of schizophrenia. She'd menstruated for the first time seven months earlier but had no periods subsequently. Her initial symptoms were consistent with manic illness—loss of sleep, excess activity, pressure to talk, and loosening of associations. She adopted the firm belief that she had been given special discounts from a local shop and began knocking on neighbors' doors, offering to buy things for them. Then, within forty-eight hours, the symptoms altered. Now she was severely depressed, cried easily, and was overcome with a sense of anguish. She clung to her mother and could not tolerate it when she left her side. These symptoms lasted two more days. Then, in another two days, all her symptoms went away and she behaved normally for twenty-two days.

Her psychosis then reappeared, lasting six days. This time she was treated with an antipsychotic drug, which reduced the overall intensity of her condition but did not fully resolve it. The pattern of six days of symptoms and twenty-two days of remission continued. While electroencephalography (a measurement of the electrical pathways in the brain) was performed twice, during her remission and during her acute phase, it proved negative, and doctors were mystified.

Her resourceful physician began to investigate the patterns of her illness and arrived at the conclusion that the psychotic episodes had actually replaced the girl's menstrual cycles. On the basis of this information, the antipsychotic medication was withdrawn, and she was treated with progesterone. After that she experienced no psychotic episodes, her periods reappeared, and she was discharged from the clinic. The young woman was fortunate that her physician considered a hormonal imbalance, since the clinical picture can often be so misleading. Patients with unusual episodic illnesses are likely to be treated as schizophrenic.

Dr. Bruce McEwen is not surprised that such crises occur, especially in a transitional period like puberty. He sees a comparison with catamenial epilepsy, a form of epilepsy that varies in frequency during the menstrual cycle. "Basically what we see with catamenial epilepsy," he explains, "is a nervous system that has reached its limit. Some of the internal systems are at the far edge of their operating range. And when you have a change in hormones which affect these systems, they can get to the point where they cause severe emotional and behavioral reactions."

But it's not just extreme cases that need to be cited. Even the normal rise and flow of estrogen during a regular menstrual cycle can affect mental performance. Young women do better on Dr. Barbara Sherwin's word-pair memory tests during the luteal phase of their cycles, when estrogen and progesterone levels are high, than during menstruation, when hormone levels are low. "This doesn't mean women are less competent late in their cycles," says Dr. Sherwin. "The changes are too minor to have any effect in the real world."

But lest one forget, the "real world" for at least a half million

young women a year revolves around such mental acuity events
as taking the Scholastic Aptitude Test. Dr. Sherwin's findings
could turn out to be a watershed where testing is concerned.
The SAT, a critical determinant for college placement, tests cognitive and analytical skills. It calls upon students to make fine
discriminations in word relationships and reading passages. It
is disturbing to think of the disadvantage young women may
experience when they take the SAT during this period of estrogen deficiency. Cyclical hormonal imbalance may be a critical
piece in assessing school behavior and performance. Dr. Toran-
Allerand explains that "estrogen exerts its influence by making
neurons more sensitive to stimulus of nerve growth factor,
wiring dendrites and axons that allow neurons to communicate
and give birth to new synapses between one neuron and another that are necessary for the mastery of new tasks and ideas."
In other words, when estrogen levels are low, there may be cognitive impairment. We need to be sensitive to the possibility that
a percentage of young women may be taking a crucial test at an
unadvantageous time. This is an area that has never been addressed by school authorities or educators. Until now, it has not
been understood.

## A Double Standard

It is likely that periodic psychosis in puberty is merely a more
severe form, or perhaps a subgroup, of PMS. If so, it should be
something that the medical community can easily understand.
Premenstrual syndrome, after all, is the only female hormone-
related illness that is officially acknowledged by the American

Psychiatric Association. In the *Diagnostic and Statistical Manual of Mental Disorders* (DSM-IV-R), premenstrual psychiatric illness is listed as a discrete organic disorder.

Although this seems to be a progressive step toward validating the real experiences of women, it is somewhat gratuitous. The problem is, if a mental disorder is not listed in the DSM-IV-R, it is said not to exist. You can't have it if it's not named! So, even while the American Psychiatric Association is encouraging treatment for premenstrual illnesses, it is perilously neglecting the unique qualities and hazards of postpartum and perimenopausal illnesses. This makes absolutely no sense. If alterations in levels of progesterone or estrogen in premenstrual syndrome cause mood disorders, how could postpartum psychiatric illness, which puts mothers and babies at tremendous risk, be ignored? Moreover, for the medical establishment to simply dismiss as midlife neurotics the millions of women who suffer from clinical depression and psychosis in the perimenopause is as incomprehensible as it is medieval. In fact, Dr. Ari Birkenfeld, associate professor of reproductive endocrinology at Mt. Sinai Hospital in New York, has affectionately designated PMS as "preparation for menopause syndrome."

The repercussions of dismissing menopausally related illnesses are devastating in their impact—not only medically but in other ways as well. Since insurance companies base decisions regarding reimbursements for treatment on the DSM-IV-R, many women may find themselves unable to afford critically needed medical care.

Although it is well known that suicide attempts and admissions to psychiatric hospitals occur more often in women premenstrually, the women who suffer from postpartum and peri-menopausal psychiatric illness experience the same range of disabling symptoms as the women who meet the diagnostic criteria for PMS. In all three conditions, the symptoms are so severe as to disrupt and, in some cases, ruin their lives. These include sleep disturbances, anxiety attacks, severe mood swings, and clinical depression.

It is clear that the brain is sensitive, in many ways, to ovarian hormones. In premenstrual, perimenopausal, and postpartum psychotic illness, the hormone imbalance has severely altered the symptom-producing threshold in predisposed women. Menopause, like all the major hormonal transitions, has the potential to produce biological problems with serious psychological manifestations, especially in highly susceptible women. Balancing our hormones is crucial to all women's sense of well-being.

Perhaps the most disturbing fact is that postpartum psychiatric illness is excluded from medical recognition. Vast numbers of psychiatrists still deny its existence, dispensing the usual bromidic disclaimers that psychiatric illness after having given birth is not significantly different from other psychiatric illnesses. The consequences of such thinking are horrifying to contemplate.

### The Postpartum Tragedy

Angela Verlyn's postpartum psychosis led to a tragedy that has grown all too common: She slit her baby's throat. Angela later described in a television interview the delusions that led to such a shocking result. "I remember picking up the knife, but I had no thought of killing my baby until I got to him," she said.

"I thought we would all go to heaven if I did it. That's when I cut his throat. My only thought was, 'God, help me do this." I was reading the Bible where Abraham sacrifices his son. I thought I would have God's favor if I did this act. I thought either my husband or the pastor would raise him from the dead if we didn't all go to heaven that day."

How is such a thing possible?

According to the *British Journal of Psychiatry,* severe postpartum psychosis may affect one in every five hundred new mothers. These women experience terrifying delusions and hallucinations. There is personality change; mood swings occur very quickly. Sometimes voices are heard; sometimes there are overwhelming impulses. This is not a new phenomenon; the syndrome was described by Hippocrates and again by Galen in the earliest medical treatises. In the fifteenth century the first detailed clinical history of a postpartum case emerged, in an autobiography dictated by the patient herself, Margery Kempe of Lynn, England. Married to a wealthy former member of Parliament, Margery gave birth to a child and became psychotic a few days later. The psychosis took the form of hallucinations, delusions, and violent expression around a religious theme. She exhibited a strong urge to visit religious centers and attend ceremonies—an urge in which she was indulged by her husband. In such places she was often seized by disruptive bursts of crying and screaming. Recurrences followed several pregnancies, with a similar pattern of explosive outbursts of religious fervor during the late phase of the illness.

Doctors have long believed that postpartum psychiatric illness is related to the sharp decline in estrogen that occurs immediately after childbirth. Estrogen levels normally fluctuate from 80 to 200 picograms per liter of blood in women of reproductive age who are not pregnant. During pregnancy the levels shoot up to 5,000 picograms, and immediately after childbirth they plummet to the range of 80 to 100 picograms. Studies show a relationship between the hormone and several neurotransmitters that influence mood, including serotonin.

According to Dr. James Hamilton, America's leading expert on postpartum disorders, if one stands back and looks at the broad picture of postpartum psychiatric illness, a rather simple pattern becomes apparent. There are two severe disorders that appear after childbirth. The first is an agitated, volatile, psychosis that begins after three days and has a peak incidence of onset on the sixth day. The psychosis may end abruptly or extend into months of confusion or depression, a state sometimes interrupted by a violent episode of psychotic thinking and behavior. The second severe disorder develops insidiously after the second or third week, has predominant depressive features, and often is associated with physical complaints, sometimes signs that are similar to those seen in thyroid deficit.

Dr. Hamilton explains that women who experience postpartum psychosis are not losing their minds; they are responding in some way to changes in their bodies. He says that "during pregnancy, the placenta, the organ that controls the flow of nourishment to the fetus, acts as a hormone factory, producing as much as ten times the normal amount of hormones like progesterone and estrogen. After childbirth, with the loss of the placenta, the mother's body must resume manufacturing hormones on its own at the proper levels. In some cases there is a delayed reaction, resulting in a hormone deficit which can affect brain chemistry."

Dr. Hamilton believes that the endocrine deregulation that occurs during the postpartum period is set in motion by three major events. The first is delivery of the fetus and placenta, which removes a large source of hormone production. The second is the withdrawal of estrogen, which leads to lowering serum-binding protein and lower serum levels of many of the circulating hormones. The third change is the elevation of prolactin, a potent inhibitor of many endocrine functions that occurs with delivery and with breast-feeding. Thus the sudden postpartum fall of estrogen may be the first step in a sequence of events involving the endocrine system that provoke symptoms of serious psychiatric disorder in susceptible individuals. Infanticide and suicide are two catastrophic outcomes of postpartum psychiatric illness.

"There was a time when we thought people with epilepsy were possessed by the devil," says the psychologist Dr. Susan Hickman, "and then we learned that this was a disorder of the brain. This illness, postpartum psychosis, is just as much a biochemical disorder of the brain as diabetes or epilepsy."

Understanding that her actions were influenced by biochemical changes in her brain is small consolation for Sheryl Massip. This twenty-six-year-old mother killed her six-week-old baby in the grip of postpartum psychosis. Although Sheryl had been suffering both visual and auditory hallucinations for weeks before the killing, no one had paid the slightest attention—until the day she walked into the middle of a busy street with her child and flung him in front of an oncoming car. The car swerved, and the baby survived. Before anyone could react, Sheryl grabbed the baby from the street, took him into a garage next to her house, and smashed his brains in with a wrench. Sheryl then got into her car and drove over her baby's head. Getting out of the car, Sheryl picked up her baby, cradled him in her arms, and started walking down the street. A police officer would later report, "We could trace her path by the brains and blood drippings."

Amazingly, Sheryl managed to escape detection. She dumped the baby in a trash can and returned home. She arrived covered with blood and told her husband that a black woman in a red wig had come up to her and snatched the baby out of her arms. Sheryl was arrested soon after and charged with murder.

At her trial Sheryl's attorney entered a plea of not guilty by reason of insanity, but the jury found her sane and announced a verdict of guilty of second-degree murder.

The judge, however, announced that he was compelled to overturn the jury's verdict. In light of the evidence as he saw it, the judge ruled that although Sheryl had killed her child she did not commit murder. He declared that she was insane, suffering from postpartum psychosis. His ruling created a precedent in the state of California.

Other countries are more progressive. The Parliament of Great Britain, for example, passed the Infanticide Act in 1922. The act rests on the premise that there is a direct relationship between childbearing and a resulting mental illness. If a mother in Great Britain kills her child within the first year of its life, she is charged not with murder but instead with the reduced charge of manslaughter.

The United States has been slow to recognize the extent of postpartum illness. In the late 1980s, Lorenza Penguella was put on trial for a crime that shocked San Diego, California. In September 1986, Lorenza had wandered the waterfront docks for hours, her five-month-old baby, Sara, bundled snugly in her arms. At one point Lorenza stopped a passing woman and begged her to take the child; she offered to give her baby away. The woman rebuffed her and fled. The baby's corpse was found floating in San Diego Harbor the next morning. Lorenza was arrested, jailed, and charged with murder.

The police psychiatrist who interviewed Lorenza was shaken by the encounter. "This poor woman shouldn't have been in jail. She needed to be under proper treatment in a hospital. I couldn't believe the situation. She was in a full-blown psychotic state. She thought there were rats all over her. She tried to set herself on fire. She desperately needed help. Instead, she's in a jail cell. They're not treating her at all."

The case against Lorenza Penguella never advanced to a trial. Instead, she plea-bargained to a lesser charge of manslaughter and was sentenced to four years in prison. But her psychiatrist was distressed with the result, believing that prison is no solution for women who have committed crimes while under the influence of postpartum psychosis.

"If they believe they're killing a rat and they don't see their child, they see a rat," he observed. "That's their experience of it; it's not some game. These women never intend to kill their children. If they were okay, if they were normal, they'd be more horrified than *we* are. We must still be in the Dark Ages to throw people into prisons when we should be putting them in hospitals and helping them."

There is usually little compassion for a mother who kills her child. The cultural taboo against infanticide is so powerful that the enormity of such a crime overwhelms normal emotions. Human sympathy goes only so far. Yet it may be a tragic mistake to portray such women as willful murders. If there are extenuating circumstances—a chemical or hormonal imbalance that has created severe psychotic reactions—then these women should be placed under a physician's care and treated. Instead, they are put on trial for murder, found guilty, and imprisoned.

The Oregon Regional Primate Research Center studies, cited by Dr. Peter Kramer in *Listening to Prozac*, may have relevance to postpartum aggression. "Because rhesus monkeys are naturally aggressive within the species, they were chosen for large-scale studies on the relationship between serotonin and aggression," Kramer writes. "The monkeys' spinal fluid was tested for levels of a serotonin-breakdown product, or metabolites. High aggressivity correlated with low levels of the metabolites, a sign of low brain-serotonin levels.

"Studies indicate that humans are similar to monkeys in this regard. In human children and adolescents, low levels of a serotonin metabolite in the spinal fluid predict the severity of physical aggression on follow-up two and a half years later."

If these findings prove true, then the Oregon Primate Studies become a flashpoint for broader investigation into the role of estrogen in triggering psychiatric illness. The work in the Oregon studies was in the brain stem in the rafe nucleus, which not only contains the cell body, but all the machinery for running the cell. Thus the Oregon primate research was done at the primary site in the brain and results are compelling.

The studies show that estrogen works on the cell bodies of the mid-brain rafe neurons to increase the tryptophane enzyme that *produces* serotonin. Estrogen deprivation dramatically lowers the levels of serotonin in the brain. In a study of 123 women in separate trials, low blood tryptophan was linked to maternity blues. (Handley et. al. 1977 and 1980)

If the form of aggression in the rhesus monkey is a model for human violence against the self or family members, as studies suggest, it may also be a perfect model to understand postpartum psychotic depression by providing an explanation for the unspeakable crimes of mothers against their own offspring.

These studies clearly raise some important issues surrounding the need for short-term estrogen replacement in postpartum women, almost as routine therapy. The drop in estrogen levels is so abrupt and the ability to determine which women are predisposed to psychiatric illness is so uncertain, that not administering estrogen may be putting women at unnecessary risk.


My emotional state during my own breakdown corresponded perfectly with that of Angela Thompson, a young mother who drowned her baby in the bathtub. "I became preoccupied with religion," she said. "I felt called upon to perform this tremendous act of faith. There was a power in me. It was compelling me. I needed to express my faith in God. When a delusional state of mind takes over, you can't control what you're thinking. You're convinced that whatever you believe is real."

# 6

## *Marcia:*
## Intervention!

I was in search of a center, struggling for my balance. The world I had created was a phantasmagoric wonder, churning with experiences that propelled me forward and backward in time. In the midst of this I was never more alive, yet never closer to death. My thoughts were caught in a whirlpool, and I was trapped by their dizzying speed. It required all my strength to keep from being swept away by the madness that consumed me.

While this was happening, I was convinced that the madness would never end, that it was just the beginning of a long, dark road. And if the road *did* end, I was sure that it would end only in my death.

On this particular morning, as I set myself on automatic pilot for the drive to school, I could not have anticipated that I would reach a turning point later that day at a posh Manhattan restaurant.

The seeds for my survival had been sown more than two decades earlier in an eleventh-grade English class, when a gifted young woman named Ellen was my student. Not only had Ellen and I stayed in touch but our friendship had grown stronger over the years. Earlier that week Ellen had invited me to Lutèce to celebrate my fiftieth birthday. I know that for a lot of women turning fifty is traumatic, but I felt upbeat and optimistic. I thought I had weathered the years quite well. But I would eventually discover that my future well-being depended upon that evening.

I remember only the charm and the intimacy of that dinner. Months later Ellen would reveal that the whole experience was deeply disturbing. She told me that, throughout the evening, I seemed to be sending her urgent subliminal messages. These messages, she said, were too fast for her mind to interpret but real enough for her to feel terrified for me.

"You looked lovely that night," Ellen recalled, "and you seemed to be in such high spirits. But every once in a while—in the midst of some other topic of conversation entirely—you'd say, in a matter-of-fact way, 'God told me . . . but don't tell anyone.' Then you'd laugh it off and pick up the last thread of our conversation. At first, I wasn't even sure that you'd said what I thought you had. There was one moment when you smiled rather sadly and said quietly, 'You must really think I've lost my mind.' Then you shook your head and began talking about some new film you wanted to see. It seemed too minor at the time to make a big deal of, so I just decided to let it go."

Ellen had always been a delicate balance of strength and vulnerability. She was attuned to the subtlest shifts in the climate surrounding her relationships; that sensitivity, combined with her impassioned sense of loyalty, endowed Ellen with uncanny empathy and fairness.

What would have happened if I had dropped Ellen off at her apartment that evening and gone straight home? It was only after I accepted Ellen's invitation to come up for coffee that the magnitude of my illness became alarmingly clear to her. Once we were in her apartment, I was seized with an overwhelming desire to use the Ouija board. Of course I had it with me; I couldn't go anywhere without it by then. I convinced Ellen to use it with me. Using the Ouija board had been my unconscious purpose from the moment Ellen asked me in for coffee.

She and I sat down opposite each other in her living room. I opened the board and put it on the coffee table between us. I extended my hand and placed it on the laminated surface. Ellen's hand joined mine. As soon as our fingers touched the triangular pointer, it came alive and pulled our hands across the board in all directions. The letters flashed through the clear plastic teardrop like Chinese brushstrokes, visible one second and gone the next. My mind just as quickly recorded the words that formed. Before I could stop myself, they leapt from my mouth. I heard my voice intoning the words in a deeper register than I had ever used before: "Ellen, this is God speaking."

Ellen barked a laugh in shocked surprise, but it was short-lived. She suddenly realized that I had opened a crack in my world to her. She remembers now that I was completely serious, transported to some other realm. Alerted suddenly to some hidden truth, but bewildered by its nature, Ellen became somber. She vividly recollects the chill that went down her spine as she looked at me. She was frightened but intent on understanding what was happening. She kept her fingers next to mine on the pointer as it continued to spin around the board, partly to humor me but also because she wanted to help me. Ellen wasn't the kind of friend who would run away because you were troubled.

I felt as if I were speaking in tongues as I watched the pointer dart relentlessly across the board. I had no ability to control what I was saying. Some other power was driving me to communicate its message.

"You're irreverent, Ellen," I intoned, "but I love you anyway." And then, in my next breath, I heard my voice urging, "Ellen, get Marcia to a psychiatrist."

I immediately protested. "That's crazy. I don't need a psychiatrist. Don't listen to Him, Ellen." A wave of nausea rose over me and crashed; I suddenly felt as if I were tottering on a fault line between two conflicting realities. My point of reference had been the Ouija board, and until this moment I had trusted it. Now it was betraying me.

Ellen ignored my plea. She was fixated on the board and refused to look at me. "You want me to take Marcia to a psychiatrist like Dr. Bloomfield out on Long Island?" she asked the board.

Our hands moved with the pointer once again. "Yes," I heard myself responding flatly, betrayed again by forces that were instructing me about what to say.

Furiously attempting to regain control, I stood up, pushed the Ouija board off the table, and said, "Forget it, Ellen. Just forget it. This is ridiculous. Let's not play this stupid game anymore."

I somehow managed to get out of Ellen's apartment and find my way home, the Ouija board still with me. I begged Ellen to forget what had happened, claimed to have a doctor's appointment already scheduled, and convinced her it was just that I had been under a lot of pressure. That was all it was, I told her—pressure.

Now, looking back on that horrible time, I think that my unconscious mind erupted in a desperate struggle with itself. The part of me that could no longer withstand living in this delusional madness was trying to destroy the part of me that refused to relinquish the Ouija board. I couldn't give it up; it had grafted itself onto my life. But my unconscious had an agenda of its own and decided to resolve the crises on its own terms.

A couple of days after my dinner with Ellen, during a long interval between classes, I slipped into one of the girls' bathrooms at school. Concealed in a stall, I eased myself down on the toilet seat and hunched over the board. As I placed my fingers gently on the pointer, it instantly flew out from under my hand, then gradually slowed, moving in bold and even strokes around the letters. And in that same moment, I heard the voice of God thundering in my mind as if He were directly over and around me:

NOW I MUST LEAVE, MARCIA. YOU WILL THROW THE BOARD AWAY ON PAIN OF DEATH.

I felt my whole body collapse in anguish. Tears poured down my face, and I began to shake and heave in sobs.

"Please," my inner voices shrieked, "please, don't leave me. Stay with me. What will I do without you?"

The pointer in my hand slowed to a deliberate and commanding rhythm. Suddenly I heard Ben's voice clearly in my mind.

YOU WILL LIVE. YOU WILL LOVE. AND YOU WILL DO GOOD DEEDS.

I clung to the gentle sound of Ben's voice. Tears streamed down my cheeks. "I love you," I cried silently.

The pointer moved again. YOU ARE LOVED, MARCIA. Then I heard what I knew to be the voice of God. NOW THROW THE BOARD AWAY.

I rocked back and forth, clutching the board against me. I sensed a sudden emptiness, the withdrawal of a powerful presence. I hugged the board and sat in silence, numbed by the insensibility that accompanies loss. I sat, waiting. The room was draped in silence. Then, slowly, like an invalid, I stood up, opened the door of the stall, and walked the few feet to the rubbish bin. I gently placed the board in the bin and buried it under mounds of paper towels.

I turned to leave, but suddenly, overcome with panic, like a lover unable to say good-bye, I reached inside the bin and retrieved the board. I stumbled into one of the stalls and latched the door. Again, I place the pointer on the surface of the board.

"Please," I whispered, sobbing now, "please come back. Please don't leave me."

Slowly I felt the pointer begin to move across the board again. It moved in almost the same commanding rhythm as the voice I could hear booming in my head. The words made me shudder with terror:

MARCIA, NOW YOU WILL DIE.

"No," I begged. "Please, I need one more chance. Give me

another chance. Please." I held my breath and waited. I felt a bolt of lightning explode all around me. My head seemed to open up, and my eyes filled with a golden light, brilliant and dazzling. I saw the word GOD flare up in enormous letters. Each letter was ablaze, incandescent and blinding. I was transfixed as they vaulted into empty space. The pointer came alive beneath my hand and gathered momentum, sliding across the board. The voice of God spoke once again. Gently this time, like a father giving his child a blessing.

NOW, GO, MARCIA. IT IS TIME TO SAY GOODBY. THROW THE BOARD AWAY FOREVER. YOU ARE LOVED. YOU ARE BLESSED.

The pointer became still. The voice was silent. I pushed the stall door open and walked toward the rubbish bin. I tunneled a hole with my hands and reburied the board under a mound of paper towels. Then I left the room. I had only one more class to teach.

Somehow I managed to make it through the next hour. With five minutes remaining in the school day, I was eager to be out of the classroom. As I turned to the board to write the assignment for the next day, I noticed my friend Joan, a guidance counselor at the school, motioning to me through the window of my door. Joan is adept at sifting through the complexities of family crises, and I had often turned to her for insight and support when one of my students was troubled. I was certain that the reason for her appearance had something to do with a student.

"Hi, what's up?" I asked, poking my head out the door.

"Before you leave today, could you stop by my office for a minute. It's important. Okay?" she asked.

"You want to see me? What for?" I was surprised that Joan would encroach on my after-school time. I attempted to beg off with some plausible excuse, but Joan had already turned to walk away, oblivious to my protest.

"Hey, wait a minute," I shouted down the hall after her. But without breaking her stride, she glanced backward and said, "It's important. Okay?"

As I stood in the doorway, the final bell sounded and the hall began to fill with students rushing to escape the confinement of the building. My students jostled me as they fled the classroom, and I was irritated and anxious. I resented Joan for intruding on my personal time. I was not in the mood for either socializing or involving myself in new problems. I needed to get out of the building, and I had a good mind to just leave. She could call me later if it were all that important. But as I was about to head down the staircase to the door leading outside, I made an abrupt turn to my right instead and walked down the hallway to Joan's office, promising myself I would stay only a minute.

But when I stepped through the doorway of her office, my indignation and whatever intentions I may have had completely vanished from my mind. I was stunned, trying to make sense out of the sight that greeted me. Standing alongside Joan's desk, their faces taut with concern, were Ellen and my friend Ruth, who is always at her best when someone is in crisis. She has a way of entering your space with intimate concentration, her presence resonating with concern and reassurance.

My eyes shifted from one to the other. I was struck with a sudden feeling of dislocation. I was confused about where they belonged, as if both women were out of uniform.

"What are you doing here?" I asked.

They seemed to fill the entire space of the already cramped office, and I was aware of a growing sense of panic. I detected a trace of smugness in their manner. I felt as if I were being patronized in some way, as if they knew something I didn't. There was even a condescending edge to Ruth's voice when she spoke. "We're here because we love you, Marcia," she said. "You've been a wonderful friend, and we think you're in a lot of pain."

Frightened, I slowly backed away from them until I felt myself leaning against a filing cabinet angled into a corner of the room. I knew I was in danger, and I needed to put all my energy into making myself inaccessible.

"I don't understand," I said, shaking my head furiously. "I don't know what you're doing here. Leave me alone. You had no right in coming."

"We knew if we did this by phone, you'd ignore us," Ellen said, with a note of apology in her voice. "We felt we had to come here in person. We're here because we want to help you."

"There's a doctor waiting for your call," Ruth said. "He has an appointment scheduled for you first thing in the morning, but you have to call to confirm it." She offered me a slip of paper she was holding in her hand. "Here's the number. Why don't you call him now?" But I shoved her hand away.

"There's nothing wrong with me, I told you." I was wild with resentment. I knew I had to get out of there. I knew that Ellen, Joan, and Ruth must have understood my indignation, but they could not have imagined the depths of my despair. I felt that I had been betrayed by everyone.

Ruth moved closer to me and put her arm around me, but I

pulled away. "Marcia," she said, her face filled with compassion, "do you remember what Ben used to say?"

She was looking at me with an intensity that engaged my full attention. Perhaps it was Ben's name that had so alerted me. "Remember Ben used to love saying that if three people tell you that you're dead, you had better lie down? Well, there are three of us here. What do you say? Will you make the call?"

As I looked deeply into the faces of my friends, I realized that there was nothing left I could appeal to. Ruth handed me the slip of paper with the psychiatrist's office number, and while the three of them watched in guarded silence, I made the call confirming an appointment for the following day.

"There, are you satisfied?" I said, not waiting for an answer. "Now, if you don't mind, I have to go to work. I have a class to teach this evening. You'll have to excuse me." But as I turned to leave, Joan said "Marcia, why don't you spend the night at my house, instead of traveling home so late?"

"Thanks, anyway," I said grudgingly, "but I want to sleep in my own bed."

And even though I was aware of the three women standing there, knowing that two of them had traveled a long distance and at their personal inconvenience to reach out to me, there was nothing more I wanted to say.

"I'll see you," I said, and walked out the door.

It wasn't until months later that I learned what had precipitated this meeting. Ellen, alarmed by my behavior with the Ouija board the night we'd had dinner, had told her own therapist about it the following morning. The therapist said, "You had better get your friend help while she's still able to make a therapeutic alliance with a psychiatrist. Otherwise, the voice may tell her to do something that could put her life in danger." Armed with that information, Ellen had immediately called Ruth.

It was past ten o'clock in the evening when I headed north on the Cross Island Parkway in the direction of Fort Lee. The day had seemed endless, and I was anxious to be home. Ahead I could see the George Washington Bridge outlined against the sky, its lights glistening from steel cables that swept upward into the night. As I continued along the highway, my windows opened, the breeze coming in off the water filled my head with crisp, clean air. A feeling of abandon swept over me. In a mood of reckless self-absorption, I pressed my foot down harder on the accelerator, buoyed by the rhythm of my car as it sped along the deserted highway.

But then something happened to me. As my car neared the ramp leading to the bridge, I was seized with a mounting terror. I sensed that in the surrounding darkness some signal was triggering danger. Almost immediately the image of my apartment terrace rose up in my mind. It seemed in that moment as if my terrace, not the bridge, were stretched before me, invisibly suspended in space. I felt it pulling me forward at greater and greater speed to a point where I knew I would pitch forward into the enveloping blackness and disappear forever.

I felt as if I were being sucked into a dark hole, as if my lungs were being violently squeezed. I struggled for air. In that split second, I wrenched the wheel to the right and sped onto the service road, exiting the parkway. Pulling my car over to the side of the road, I turned off the engine with shaking hands and sat shivering in the darkness. Even here I could not rid myself of the feeling of being swept into space.

In some fortuitous happening, my mind had exploded in a burst of realization that there were forces in me propelling me to my own destruction. For just one moment, I had been able to glimpse the madness that had gripped my mind, and I knew with absolute certainty that if I returned home to my apartment, I would throw myself off the terrace. It was an irresistible force, unlike any I had ever experienced. But in that instant, the dark curtain had been briefly lifted, and I knew I had to get to a safe place, a protected area. I turned the key in the ignition and began to drive back in the direction from which I had just come. In spite of my adamant refusal earlier, I knew I had to return to Great Neck and spend the night at Joan's house after all. Somewhere among the tangled jungle of synapses in my brain, a lone spark had suddenly and inexplicably activated, triggering the master switch for my survival.

# 7

## *Marcia:*
## The Search for Answers

My friends had joined together to help me, and when I regained control of my senses, I would be forever grateful for their compassion and love. But as I prepared for my appointment with Dr. Ralph Wharton, I was filled with anxiety. At that point I was still living in fear of forces that I was convinced could overpower me at any time. I wasn't sure what was going to happen next, what would be demanded of me. Everything seemed too complex, too paradoxical. I needed a lifeline to pull me back into control, but I was apprehensive about entering therapy. Was I submitting to yet another force against which I had no control? Would I become trapped in a relationship where I would always be the one in need, the supplicant in an eternal quest for balance? I needed Dr. Wharton to be an ally. Together, I hoped, we could widen the distance between my nightmare and my life. I lived in constant fear of a sudden eruption in my mind, and I needed the security of his office.

I also needed a genuine human relationship, no matter what the parameters. I flung myself completely into treatment and within weeks, it was apparent that my psychiatrist had become an important presence in my life. It came to me in a dream.

I was standing on the edge of a grassy river bank holding in my arms a large silver platter piled high with mounds of exotic fruits and cakes. As I stood there, I felt the presence of a man behind me in the shadows. I waited, my arms outstretched, laden with delicacies. Then, suddenly, on the opposite shore, Ben appeared. We looked across the river at one another for some moments, even while I was aware of the other figure, vigilant, behind me. Then I spoke softly in a voice deep with longing, "I'm sorry, Ben. I can't come across the river and feed you anymore. I'm not allowed to."

This was to be the first of many dreams which would reveal the conflicting unconscious forces from which I was struggling to free myself.

While I had yet to discover that the solution to my delusionary breaks would be found not in the world of analysis but in that of biology, I came to appreciate over time that my psychiatrist was the key who unlocked the door to my recovery. He kept me intact and alive while we both searched for the answer to my problems. And it was Dr. Wharton who ultimately directed me to Dr. Edward Klaiber, who was completely attuned to my symptoms and who became my mentor during my years of research and discovery.

In my first session with Dr. Wharton, I described my experiences with the Ouija board and the voices. He listened quietly, with a sympathetic attitude. He offered little comment, and I began to feel vulnerable and exposed. I needed to know what he was thinking. I felt that I was fighting for my life. I was trying to regain what I felt my breakdown had cost me, and more. I wanted to recover my spirit, my passion for life. His quiet face felt like an accusation.

Finally, frustrated by Dr. Wharton's silence, I exploded, half-rising out of my chair. "No matter what goes on here, you're not going to get rid of Ben. His spirit has survived, I know it. I will never give up my belief that he's communicating with me," I cried. "Never. I don't care what you think."

I was aware that my entire belief system was threatened in Dr. Wharton's presence. I believed that the voices existed. I heard them. How could they not be genuine? A big part of me was absolutely convinced that there was nothing wrong. What was happening was real. Ben was dead, but his consciousness had survived. He was communicating with me. It seemed foolish to think that Dr. Wharton was going to be able to cure me by making reality disappear.

Dr. Wharton looked at me steadily. "It doesn't matter what I think," he said quietly. "And it doesn't matter whether I believe it or not. The only thing that concerns me is how you handle it."

Something in his tone made me relax back into my chair. His face was kind, and I could hear the honest concern in his voice. At that moment I knew that I would be able to express myself without fear of humiliation or embarrassment. He was giving me permission to confide anything I wanted, without limit or reservation. Perhaps that's why I'd erupted in the first place; I needed to shatter his silence, the calm demeanor that had made me feel examined and judged. But I had misinterpreted Dr. Wharton's behavior. It was only quiet compassion and sensitivity that motivated him.

So, despite my initial apprehension, therapy became a turning point for me. From the moment I entered treatment, it was as though a giant boulder was flung against the side of my inertia; it enabled me to break through my obsession with the Ouija board and the voices in my head: the pattern of necessity, which until the moment I entered into treatment, had ruled my life. In my work with Dr. Wharton, I struggled toward disclosure, toward some sudden illumination that would explain what had happened to me.

It was not until three weeks into therapy that I was able to face the seriousness of my illness. For the first time, I realized that I was being held together by a tenuous glue that could dissolve at any time. I had gone to the library for the express purpose of looking for information on mental illness. Although Dr. Wharton had never once mentioned the word *psychotic* or *breakdown*, I needed to see if there was a definition—a name— for what had happened to me.

My favorite library is near the school where I teach. It's designed for quiet introspection. It is set on the edge of a pond and is surrounded by trees, lush lawns, and stone bridges. I found the psychology section, built a pile of books on the carpeted floor, and sank down among them. I was looking for as much information as I could find on the sudden onset of adult psychosis.

I went through one book after another, checking indexes, reading paragraphs, glancing through pages of text, until my eyes locked on a description. At first I noticed nothing unusual about the information. Nearly all the books had said the same thing concerning the onset of schizophrenia, that "the peak time of schizophrenia is at *the end of adolescence,* which is a period of significant stress." I could hardly help feeling that this illness bore little relevance to my own situation.

But as I read further, my eyes suddenly fell on this passage: "There is a second, smaller peak time of illness in *the fourth decade,* particularly for women. It may follow divorce, or the death of a parent, child, or spouse." There it was. Fourth decade or fifth decade, what did it matter? The text detailed my illness perfectly. My eyes remained glued to the page. "Schizophrenia has been regarded as a disorder of multiple ego functions, which results in the inability of the affected individual to discriminate accurately and reliably between inner and outer reality, and to maintain a stable and cohesive internal representation of self to the outside world."

I had to remind myself to breathe. This was exactly what had happened to me! "The individual experiences persecutory and grandiose delusions. Grandiose delusions reflect an exaggerated sense of importance, power, or knowledge. . . . They may also involve a relationship or an identity with an omnipotent figure. The patient may present him or herself as persecuted on the basis of these grandiose attributes or relationships. Auditory hallucinations may offer support and reassurance, but are more often critical and insulting."

I thought of the degradations I had endured as I read that

"command hallucinations issue orders that the patient may feel obliged to obey, or be unable to resist. The individual may be so fearful of imagined consequences that he or she dares not think, feel or move. The individual may markedly withdraw from the external world and become preoccupied with an internal world or egocentric thoughts, fantasies, delusions, and hallucinations. In his or her retreat to a delusional world, the adult psychotic patient does not acknowledge that he or she is ill and in need of help."

The words rose like a giant wave and crashed against my mind. It was all there, everything that I had experienced. It detailed the most pervasive aspects of my illness. I was overwhelmed by what I was reading. Why hadn't I been institutionalized? All of the symptoms, all of the delusions, were documented in this book. I was a schizophrenic, a deranged person who should have been locked up somewhere.

I was terrified. I felt as though I were subject to a menacing force. I needed to talk to Dr. Wharton.

I had been sitting awkwardly on the library's floor for well over an hour. I grabbed one of the shelves above my head and hoisted myself up. My legs were fighting me, cramped from being folded underneath me for so long, and I steadied myself. I clutched the open book as though it were a lifeline. The book had the power to rescue me; it could explain everything.

Frantic to find a telephone, I threaded my way out of the stacks and headed toward the main aisle. Suddenly I remembered that the telephones were lined up along the wall just inside the lobby, so I hurried toward the front of the building. I could see the phone booths in the distance, but I realized that they were just beyond the main desk, and the line of people waiting to check out their books seemed endless. Reluctantly, I placed the book on one end of the counter, where I could keep it in visual range; then I exited through the metal detectors and slipped into one of the phone booths.

I sorted through my wallet to find Dr. Wharton's telephone number. If I hadn't needed to speak to him so urgently, I could have left a message on his answering machine to phone me later in the evening. But that would have taken too long. I dialed the number he'd made available in case of an emergency.

By the time I heard his voice, I was frantic. "I have to see you. Please, Dr. Wharton. It's urgent." I started rambling on about the book and my illness, but he gently interrupted my monologue. "I'm sorry," he said. "I don't have any time. I'm scheduled to see patients all afternoon."

"What about tomorrow?" I asked desperately. "Can you see me tomorrow?" It was more of a plea than a question.

"Well, all right, I can see you at the hospital. Is that okay?" Whatever he had said would have been okay.

When I walked into Dr. Wharton's office at the hospital the next morning, I took a seat in front of his desk.

He leaned toward me from his chair, his eyes full of concern. "What were you saying about a book?" He was looking at the textbook I was holding in my lap. I handed it to him. He glanced at the cover and then said, casually, "I don't know this book. Tell me what has upset you."

"I was sick. I was very sick," I said, afraid that nothing had changed, and that I was still sick.

Dr. Wharton smiled at me calmly. "Yes, you were," he said quietly. "But you're much better now."

"I don't know if that's true!" I cried. "This book describes me as a full-blown schizophrenic. From what I understand, I should have been institutionalized. I'm scared. I could have another breakdown at any time."

Ignoring the book, Dr. Wharton leaned back in his chair, his eyes bright, his voice steady, and said, "Tell me what was different about your illness."

"I never stopped working," I said. "I was still able to teach."

"That's right." He seemed genuinely pleased with my response. "And what else was different?"

"I always cared about how I looked," I responded.

"That's exactly right," he said, in a tone that lifted my spirits. "And that's a big difference. A very important difference." Then he asked quietly, "Now, what else are you worried about?"

I felt my body go limp, and suddenly tears began streaming down my face. "That I will use up all my sick days from work, like today, and have another breakdown, and end up hospitalized without any income."

"That's not going to happen," he said with the assurance of a physician who has just read an X ray. "Use whatever sick days you need. It's nothing for you to worry about."

By the time I left Dr. Wharton's office, I felt tremendously relieved. He had reduced my terror by helping me to gain insight into my illness, thereby allowing me the distance that I needed in order to strengthen my mind and my heart. He also helped me to realize that I had misdiagnosed my condition. I may have suffered from an acute psychotic episode, but I was never schizophrenic. While all schizophrenics exhibit psychotic symptoms, such as delusions, hallucinations, and withdrawal from the external world, not every psychotic experience should be labeled schizophrenia. I was chastened by the fact that self-diagnosis, like self-medication, can be an extremely hazardous undertaking.

My sense of relief was short-lived, however, as I now understand it was destined to be. As long as I was in Dr. Wharton's presence, I felt solid and connected. But, left to my own devices, I would rapidly feel overpowered by thoughts and impulses I was unable to control.

Just weeks after I had entered treatment with Dr. Wharton, I awoke on a Sunday morning in Stockbridge with an overpowering urge to hang myself. To this day I can't understand this macabre fixation. If I were to consciously plan my death, I would never choose hanging. The idea of suffocating or choking or being hurt in some way has always frightened me. If I was serious about committing suicide, my method of choice would be barbiturates. But I was transfixed by the image of myself, a rope knotted around my neck, dangling from the ceiling.

I felt as if I were sealed in an airtight container, with everything else blackened out except that image of myself. And no matter how hard I tried to think of something else, to concentrate totally on some other thing, I could not erase the image from my mind. It was so compelling that I sprang from my bed, hoping the sheer movement of my body would shake my mind free from the horrifying spectacle that had grabbed me.

But the image remained. The only way I could save myself was to get out of the house. I grabbed my sweatshirt off the chair, slid into my jeans and sneakers, and fled the room by way of the glass doors that led to the lower deck. I raced down the driveway and out onto a long stretch of dirt road. I pushed my body, trying to outdistance myself. I thought if I ran fast enough I could get away from the image of my lifeless body hanging from the beams. No. The image was intact.

Then in midflight, I suddenly stopped running and stood still on the deserted road, gasping for air and listening to the pounding of my heart. Dense woods rose up on each side of me. I fought for my breath and tried to clear my mind. Again, the image of myself hanging from a rafter took hold. There seemed to be no escaping it. In desperation, I turned and ran back toward the house. I knew there was only one way I could fight this. I entered the house and returned to my bedroom, picked up the phone, and dialed Dr. Wharton's emergency number in New York. It was only seven in the morning when I reached his answering machine. In spite of the feeling that I was helplessly caught in some gravitational force field, the right words seemed to stick in my throat. I struggled; what message could I leave? Finally, I managed to say that I was in serious trouble and I needed to talk to him as soon as possible. As I waited for his call, I agonized. What words do you use? How do you broach the subject? "Please help me. I have this overpowering need to hang myself." I rehearsed alternatives in my mind as I paced back and forth. Yet, when the phone rang and it was at last my chance to speak, I said almost exactly that.

"Dr. Wharton, I see myself hanging from the beams in the house," I blurted out. "I can't stop it, I can't get the image out of my mind."

"Don't you have any self-discipline? Are you always so self-indulgent?"

I was stunned by his words. I could not comprehend their meaning. I shook my head in disbelief. What did this have to do with self-discipline or self-indulgence?

"I don't understand," I said. "What are you saying to me?"

"We'll talk about it tomorrow," he replied firmly. "We have an appointment tomorrow afternoon. I will see you in my office and we can talk about it then." And with those words, our conversation ended. Dr. Wharton had hung up.

I sat for some time with the phone in my hand, my head reeling. I had no idea what he was talking about when he said that I had no self-discipline. Why would he accuse me of being self-indulgent? And why would I want to hang myself? I put my hands over my face and pressed against my closed eyelids. I pressed until I saw kaleidoscopic images exploding behind my eyes. I didn't want to look up at the beams. I didn't want to open my eyes. Tears welled up. I stood in the center of the room sobbing uncontrollably. Dr. Wharton's rebuke had felt like a slap in the face. Strangely, it had also robbed the image of its force and distracted me from my suicidal impulse.

For the remainder of the day and all through the drive back to Fort Lee the following morning, my thoughts were in a jumble. Whenever I felt myself yielding to the terrible forces that seemed to overpower me, I would go back over my conversation with Dr. Wharton. His accusations had stung me, and I was furious. My appointment could not come soon enough.

I stormed into his office. I had barely sat down when I demanded, "What did you mean yesterday? I didn't understand what you were saying to me. You were speaking in non sequiturs."

Dr. Wharton looked at me with a glint in his eye. "Were they?" he asked, seeming surprised. "I don't remember. But we psychiatrists often speak in non sequiturs." He directed his attention toward me with such sincerity that I didn't know what else to say. We moved on to other matters, but over the next few days my thoughts of hanging myself gradually disappeared, until finally they were gone.

A horrible crisis had been averted, but as the months went by there were others. I still felt out of sorts, and I couldn't seem to predict or control the swings of emotion I had become increasingly vulnerable to. Sparks seemed to flare into wildfires, my moods seesawing between black depressions and lightning manic surges.

And for good measure, I felt rotten physically as well, which did nothing to help my moods. For the first time in my life I was having trouble sleeping, and I was completely exhausted. My skin felt so sensitive that a friend's hug made me wince. My periods were sporadic, and I was suffering from terrible pressure in my lower abdomen. But I was so concentrated on my therapy, so desperate to fix what seemed wrong with my *mind,* that I managed to ignore the promptings of my *body.* How ironic that seems now!

As the winter break approached, I began thinking that a trip overseas might distract me from my problems and act as a tonic to my flagging spirits. But I couldn't bring myself to make the reservations. Every time I was ready to pick up the phone and call a travel agent, my thoughts turned to Dr. Wharton. I didn't relish the thought of leaving the New York area for any length of time, as my security had become grounded in my psychiatrist's office. I knew it wasn't healthy to trade one obsession for another. But the idea of Dr. Wharton being out of reach filled me with so much anxiety that it seemed futile to plan on going anywhere.

Yet I was determined to take another stab at self-sufficiency. And finally I was able to complete the arrangements. Feeling satisfied with myself, I triumphantly announced to Dr. Wharton that I was spending my February vacation in London.

He never gave me any indication that he was alarmed by my decision to go abroad. When I told him about my plan, his response was, "Well, good. You're ready for some adventure."

The week before I was scheduled to leave he asked me if I would like to record our session. I had often talked to him about how I spent most of my travel time in the car listening to old tapes of Ben's radio program, *The Music of Israel,* which he had hosted for ten years. I had kept all the cassettes, and they soothed and uplifted me. However, the idea of taping my therapy sessions with Dr. Wharton had never come up before.

"Have you ever done this with anyone else?" I asked.

"No," he admitted, "but Ben's tapes seem to have helped you in the past."

"But if you don't believe in taping sessions, why do it now?" I persisted.

He said, simply, "I do whatever will help my patients."

Three hours before my trip to England, we taped our final session. As I rode to the airport in the backseat of a cab, I was overcome with sadness. I knew I'd be seeing Dr. Wharton as soon as I returned, but I couldn't ignore the sense of loss that I was experiencing.

As I boarded the aircraft, I could feel icy tendrils of fear beginning to grip me, threatening to sabotage my plans. On the surface, I was rational and calm. I was a woman on holiday having a perfectly ordinary experience. But I could sense underlying pressures beginning to build. They filled me with dread. The forces that had controlled me before were welling up once again. My thoughts kept returning to Dr. Wharton. I closed my eyes and imagined the familiarity of his office, and the comfort and safety it offered.

I was so glad that we'd taped our session. I believed that as long as I had the tape player, Dr. Wharton's encouraging words on the cassette would be able to sustain me. I was wrong.

Alone in a hotel room in the center of London I experienced fully—for the first time—the impact of Ben's death. Moments after I checked in and stepped across the threshold of my room, I was seized with a terrible sense of emptiness. It felt as if all these months I had been carrying myself around like so much dead weight. Everything began to reel in front of me, and I slipped into another dimension. I stood in the doorway, my eyes roaming back and forth. I was carefully searching each corner of the room, expecting something to rise up and attack me. In a rush of panic I tore across the room, grabbed the telephone, and dialed the hotel switchboard. I began fumbling through my wallet for Dr. Wharton's appointment card. There was hysteria in my voice that was impossible to contain when I gave the hotel operator his number.

I put the receiver back in its cradle as the operator placed the call. Time became an adversary in my desperate need to connect. I sat rigidly on the edge of the bed, staring at the phone, willing it to ring. When it finally did, I leapt to my feet as I picked it up.

"I'm sorry," the operator reported, "but we are unable to place your call. We have not been able to reach Dr. Wharton." I felt a deep ache spread through me, as though I'd been kicked in the stomach.

"Please call back and have them page him," I tried to say calmly. It must have come out somewhere between a cry and a command. I was aware of the growing panic in my voice, but I was unable to control it.

I slammed the receiver down and flung myself into a chair, hunched over in a need to contain myself. I was crazed with fear. Within moments the phone rang again, and it was Dr. Wharton. The second I heard his voice, I felt safe.

"What's happening? What's going on?" he asked, sounding worried. His concern released an outpouring of emotion in me.

"I want to come home," I cried into the phone. "Ben's dead. You're dead. And I should have died in September." I tried to control the sobs wracking my body. "My life is finished. It's over."

"You're right. Ben is dead," he said quietly, lingering over his words. "But you're alive and I'm alive. And your life is not over. Not from where I'm sitting it's not."

His words were measured. There was a coaxing quality to the way he spoke to me, calm and reassuring. The words hung on with a kind of intensity, as if he were taking a long distance reading of me or trying to anticipate his next move from far away. I had no way to know what he might have been thinking, but he was playing to the rhythm of my deepest need.

"Look, you can come home if you want to," he reassured me. "You can take a taxi to the airport and grab the next plane back. But I have a better suggestion. Why don't you have a good dinner? Then, take what I prescribed to help you sleep. Tomorrow, after you've had breakfast, give me a call. If you want to come home in the morning, then you will."

His words brought me back to reality. Dr. Wharton was right. By the time we said good-bye to each other, I felt relaxed and relieved. I remained in London, and my trip became an important turning point in my illness. It was there that I finally said farewell to my beloved Ben. I had crossed an ocean and survived.


While menopause never once occurred to me as the cause of my illness, I instinctively knew, after my return from London, that there was still something wrong with me—something that had nothing to do with my head. I believe that I could have handled the loss of Ben and other events in my life without having a breakdown—if not for menopause. It became clear to me that even though my psychological condition had become more stable thanks to my work with Dr. Wharton, the physical symptoms that had been plaguing me for some time continued unabated.

Only later would I discover that it was estrogen deprivation that had pushed me over the edge. Estrogen would prove to be the missing link—the essential element—in my story.

# 8

## *Marcia:*
## Naming the Madness

With Dr. Wharton's help, I had survived crisis after crisis. I had finally grieved for Ben. In many ways I was growing stronger. But I was still not *myself* in some kind of essential way. That bright, happy, confident woman who could walk into a room of people with utter ease seemed only a distant memory. I still felt fragile and off center, as if at any minute I could topple back into madness.

For the most part, I kept these matters to myself. I was living and working as a stable person, all signs of shakiness invisible to those around me. My dear friends who had intervened at my time of deepest despair were delighted to witness my recovery. They often told me how much better I seemed, and I was both buoyed and unnerved by their relief.

Ironically, this plateau of mental stability only highlighted how unwell I was feeling *physically*. The symptoms that had plagued me off and on for the past year were growing worse. Now it was my body, not my mind, that seemed in crisis.

The worst moment came one afternoon as I was sitting in my car in the parking lot of an A & S department store in Manhasset, Long Island. Without warning, I experienced a tremendous pressure in my lower abdomen, and then I felt a sudden gush and my underclothing grew heavy with wetness. I was hemorrhaging. I tied my jacket around my waist and managed to get myself to the ladies' room, where I improvised a packing. Then I went to a pay phone and called my gynecologist. He told me to come right in.

Although it was a traumatic experience for me, my gynecologist didn't seem overly concerned. "These things happen sometimes." He shrugged. "Especially around the time of menopause."

As it turned out, this was to be my last menstrual period. As I reflected on the incident, it seemed momentous, coming as it did at a critical point in my therapy. It felt like a last great death cry of nature, occurring simultaneously with some deeply emotional issues that I was working on in my sessions with Dr. Wharton.

In notes I made at the time I wrote,

> I've come to feel that breakthrough bleeding is not a phenomenon occurring at the end of the menstrual cycle, but a sloughing off of the lining of the psyche, as if pieces of coagulated memory wedged their way free through crevices of the mind, triggering conscious awareness, releasing mute screams born of loss, or love, or hope.

I now see that my unconscious mind, in an extraordinary creative leap, made the connection between my mind and my body long before I could consciously articulate that the disintegration of my mind was the result of a shutting down of my ovaries and the devastating consequences of estrogen deprivation. Throughout the two-and-a-half-year interval between Ben's death and my breakdown, and throughout my early months in therapy, it had never once occurred to me that I was going through menopause and that my breakdown was in any way estrogen related.

Several weeks passed. There was no more bleeding, but my other symptoms stayed with me—the wilted sense of being without energy, the dizziness, the inability to sleep deeply no matter how tired I was. The tingling in my legs continued, too.

It became almost routine that at some point in my therapy session I would say, "There's something still wrong with me and it's not my head." I began to sense that something was physically wrong with me that was entirely separate from the emotional issues surrounding Ben's death. I was no longer willing to downplay my symptoms.

Finally, suspecting that I might have a hormonal imbalance, Dr. Wharton arranged for me to get a blood test. It was such a simple thing—a blood test. How remarkable that it would hold all the secrets to my condition.

This particular test measures the levels of follicle-stimulating hormone—FSH. Follicle-stimulating hormone is produced by the pituitary gland to stimulate the ovaries to produce estrogen. Many years before there is any hint of menopause—indeed, while menstrual cycles are normal and a woman is still fertile, the ovaries begin responding more slowly to the stimulation of FSH. As a result, the pituitary gland compensates by producing *more* FSH. The gradual slowdown in the ovaries' production of estrogen continues through perimenopause, and the pituitary continues to increase its output of FSH. By the time a woman ceases to produce estrogen, FSH levels have reached their highest level.

| | Premenopause | Perimenopause | Menopause |
|---|---|---|---|
| FSH Levels | under 30 IU/ml | 30+ IU/ml | 40+ IU/ml |

Thus, the shutdown of the ovaries not only produces an estrogen deficiency but it also produces an overactive pituitary function. Since it is the pituitary gland that regulates hormonal activity in the body, an overactive pituitary can throw everything else into chaos.

Viewing the results of my blood test, my doctor informed me that my ovaries had completely stopped producing estrogen, and my FSH levels topped 40 IU/ml. I was in menopause. He recommended that I immediately begin a course of hormone replacement. He put me on a twenty-five-day cyclical regimen—which was the conventional therapy. The first fifteen days I took only estrogen. The next ten days I took a combination of estrogen and progestin (in the form of Provera). With this combination, at the end of Day 25, the endometrial lining sloughs off and there is usually a light menstrual period.

The moment I began taking estrogen I felt as though someone had injected adrenaline into my brain. I felt my mind expanding, surging with vitality, and I experienced instantaneous well-being. But it was the tangible effects of estrogen replacement that put the final piece in place for me. All my symptoms disappeared. My skin became moist, almost glowing, the shadow above my upper lip was no longer visible, and the crawling sensations on my skin and the pressure in my lower abdomen vanished.

While I experienced many dramatic changes both physically and emotionally within the first few weeks on estrogen, one event clearly marked an important step in my recovery. It occurred early one morning as I drove along my usual route to school. There was nothing remarkable happening. But, as my hands grabbed the steering wheel, a surge of energy flowed through me. It felt like a geyser that had been divided into ribbons of water and had suddenly and dramatically fused, gushing skyward with extraordinary force. I remember how it rushed through my head, like the steady motion of a strong current, a pure stream of energy, and I experienced an extraordinary feeling of wholeness. I was ecstatic. I had become so accustomed to living a divided life, in which my inner world, ruled by lies and illusions, was more real to me than the everyday world I worked in. But somehow, inexplicably, I knew they had now merged.

It didn't seem possible that I could experience such complete wellness in mind and body from simply taking a pill. Could it be that my two and a half years of hell might have been prevented? That until the end my doctors had missed the hormonal component in my illness? I wasn't sure. Perhaps my mental illness *was* a result of delayed mourning for Ben, as Dr. Wharton had suggested. Perhaps the beginning of my estrogen treatment merely coincided with my coming to terms with my grief. In a sense, Ben's death had muddied up my diagnosis. I was seen as a traumatized widow who had lost her ability to cope, rather than a midlife woman in the throes of a hormonal balance. I would later hear from many women who had experienced the same attitudes from professionals. Doctors seemed eager to find psychosomatic reasons for mental symptoms—especially for women of a certain age:

"You just went through a traumatic divorce . . ."
"Your mother died . . ."
"You're depressed by signs of aging . . ."
"Your children have left the nest . . ."

It's all too easy to find rationales in daily life. However, I always found it odd and disturbing that doctors could so quickly reach these conclusions with women who had never before shown any signs of mental illness.

There is no mistaking the rejuvenating effects of estrogen. Symptoms seem to vanish like magic. But the issues surrounding hormone replacement are far more complicated, as I was about to discover. After some months on estrogen, I awoke on a Saturday morning seriously depressed. All I could do was to lie in bed and cry, but there was nothing tangible to account for my feelings. I called Dr. Wharton.

Our phone conversation, though brief, gave me the support I knew I would need to help me through the weekend, but when I awoke the following morning, I was shocked to discover that I was no longer depressed. In some extraordinary biological happening, my depression had vanished, and the only clue I had that could in any way account for such a phenomenon was the fact that when I had used the bathroom during the night, I discovered I was staining.

I instinctively knew there had to be some hormonal connection between the fact that I had been in the throes of a clinical depression on Saturday, on Saturday night I'd had some staining, and on Sunday morning I was overflowing with feelings of well-being.

In what would turn out to be another defining moment in my illness, Dr. Wharton suggested that I see a colleague who was doing research at the Columbia Psychiatric Institute on PMS and other hormonally related disorders.

I was impressed but unsettled by the directness of her questions. "Why did you begin treatment with Dr. Wharton?" she asked. "He didn't give me any background."

"I had an acute psychotic episode with auditory hallucinations," I answered, relaxing into the interview.

"That was probably estrogen related," she said. It seemed to me that not a moment had elapsed between my question and her answer, and I was both relieved and elated. She had confirmed what I had been suspecting for some time.

"And why has he sent you to see me now?" she asked.

"Because a week ago I became so depressed that I wanted to die. And then I had staining and I suddenly wasn't depressed anymore."

She regarded me intently for a moment and then said, without a trace of hesitation, "That sounds like Provera poisoning. You probably need to change the dosage of estrogen and Provera."

She went on to explain that hormone replacement therapy requires fine tuning—and sometimes trial and error—to find the right balance. "Each woman will have a different response to the ratio of estrogen to progesterone in her system," she said. "Your estrogen levels were not high enough to offset the high levels of progesterone. The result for you was a clinical depression—essentially an extreme form of artificially induced PMS."

Only a highly trained and experienced clinician could have grasped so effortlessly the hormonal component in my illness. My encounter with her added an important dimension to my understanding of the biochemical nature of my illness and would prompt the neuroendocrinologist Dr. Bruce McEwen to say to me some months later, "If only we had more anecdotes of this kind to help us in our research."

Dr. Wharton's colleague talked about the facility with which she was able to identify my psychotic episode as an estrogen-related illness. "We know that many women have marked mood changes in relationship to abrupt hormonal changes," she said. "For example, postpartum psychosis, premenstrual syndrome, and in menopausal estrogen replacement therapy. I've seen women suddenly become very depressed when large doses of Provera get added to their estrogen in their menopausal estrogen replacement regimen. Clinically, I have seen enough marked mood changes that were related to these hormonal states."

I had never given much thought to the role of progesterone in depression, but I would later learn that it may well be the key to understanding hormonally triggered depression. As Dr. McEwen would explain to me, "One of the problems these days is that whenever you give estrogen, people are scared because of the cancer risk. Progesterone is given as a way of reducing that risk—at least that's been the belief of the medical community. In menopause, cyclical progestins are necessary to counteract the endometrial action of the estrogens. They produce a withdrawal bleeding, but they also produce PMS-like symptoms. It may be that in many cases of PMS, progesterone is responsible for the symptoms. In fact, menopause-like hot flashes often coexist with PMS symptoms. But opposed therapy, using both estrogen and progestins in combination, is the standard treatment. The problem is that progesterone *does* oppose what estrogen does. It works that way in the brain as well as in other organs, so you are likely to undo what you are trying to achieve with estrogen."

Dr. Klaiber agreed. In his research, he told me, when severely depressed women were cycled with estrogen and progesterone, there was a marked difference in their depression according to their regimen. "When they were on estrogen, their suicidal feelings subsided, but on the progesterone, the suicidal feelings recurred. I have one patient now who's having a terrible time. She is a woman who suffers from severe perimenopausal depression, and estrogen has made a tremendous difference. But when we put her on progesterone, she becomes suicidal."

Dr. Wharton's colleague provided the missing link in my search for answers. But she also provided medical confirmation, for the first time, that my breakdown had a medical explanation. As she explained the biological changes that had triggered my depression, my spirits soared. Everything that had happened to me began to make sense. It had been the dramatic shift in the balance of my hormones that had caused my plunge into a delusional world. Without revealing any emotion to her, inwardly I was burning with frustration. I was angry at my physicians for not having considered the possibility that my symptoms were related to perimenopause. But at the same time, I was ecstatic, and overflowing with relief. She had confirmed what, at some level, I had suspected all along. While menopause had never crossed my mind as the cause of my illness, within weeks of beginning therapy with Dr. Wharton, I instinctively knew that there was something wrong with me that had nothing to do with my head. Everything in my own experience indicated that I could have handled the events in my life without severe trauma. It was also evident to me that even though my psychological condition had become more stable, my physical symptoms continued unabated. It was estrogen deprivation that had put me over the edge. Not only did she know what had happened to me but, more important, she knew why.

Her insights provided an entirely new dimension to my breakdown, which seems to me now to have been the ultimate example of "body language." Biological forces were driving me, charging my brain, and since my mind could not withstand the terrible insults of my body, it had short-circuited. The collapse of my mind coincided with the shutting down of my ovaries. It was a simultaneous disintegration of my mind and my body.

In his book *The Mismeasure of Man,* the evolutionary biologist Stephen Jay Gould writes, "Humans are animals, and everything we do is constrained, in some sense, by our biology. Some constraints are so integral to our being that we rarely even recognize them, for we never imagine that life might proceed another way." This is uniquely true for women who, throughout their perimenopausal years, have been so battered by the emotional and physical stress of the biochemical changes in their bodies that their feelings of self-worth have been crushed. They are not only "brain weary," but "life weary" and since they have no understanding of the biological causes of their illness, often blaming themselves, they see no way that things can ever change. Without the right kind of intervention, they may be lost.

If any perimenopausal tragedy points up the need for such therapeutic intervention, it is that of Christine's, who I came across while doing my research. After multiple attempts at suicide, a diagnosis of manic-depressive illness, institutionalization, lithium, and a dozen shock therapy treatments, the discovery that Christine was not only perimenopausal but seriously estrogen deficient turned her life around.

"My psychiatrist finally sent me to an endocrinologist," she said. "It changed everything for me. He said that hormonally I was a total mess, my numbers were everywhere. I was definitely perimenopausal, and he put me on estrogen replacement. He told me that he had never seen such a change in a person as he has seen in me since I've been on estrogen.

"When I first saw him I was very shaky, very frightened, very meek, very weepy, very fragile. But after I started taking the estrogen, I was outgoing. I don't think it changed my personality. It wasn't like Prozac or anything like that. But my head was clearer. I could think. I could function. It was amazing. I didn't realize there was such a difference. I couldn't sense the change because it was so gradual that it wasn't that obvious to me, but other people could see it. When I saw my doctor once a month and then once every other month, he noticed tremendous changes in the way I walked, the way I carried myself, the way I spoke."

But it hasn't been a totally smooth transition for Christine. The tragedy of a misdiagnosis like Christine's is the way it warps relationships—sometimes destroying them forever. Recently, Christine and her husband separated.

"I believe my husband was really threatened by the new me, by the change in my personality," she mused. "He may have wanted me to be that weak, helpless, dependent woman, and when I became my own person, he couldn't enjoy it and grow with it. He couldn't enjoy me. I became more outspoken, more assertive, expressed my likes and dislikes. It was a second marriage, full of promise, and it just came unraveled. But I can't let myself obsess about it. What I need to do now is get my life straightened out.

"I've been living for so many years feeling isolated and alone. I'm still living with it. But therapy is helping me get back on my feet to see who I am. To see how I'm valued as a person. What I'm finding more difficult than anything is getting rid of my old habits. Even though I feel better and my thinking is better, my old day-to-day habits are still there; they've been so conditioned over the years, and I have to remember to change them. What I do and what I say is not what I mean anymore. It's like I'm out of sync. My responses are so automatic. I have to undo that, but I know it will take time."

Therapy is helping Christine process her new perceptions so that she is no longer a woman divided from herself. It is helping her become more in tune with her thinking, and integrate what she feels with what she does. She'll make it. But I can't help feeling terribly sad when I encounter women like Christine. All they've been through is such a waste, and it never had to happen.

# 9

# The Great Estrogen Debate

A couple of years after I started taking estrogen, Mary, a close friend of mine in her late forties, began describing symptoms that seemed all too familiar—inexplicable panic attacks, strange tingling sensations, a sudden fear that people were staring at her and judging her. She grew convinced that her boss was planning to fire her—which wasn't true—and imagined that he was watching her every move—also not true. I'd known Mary for years, and all this was completely out of character for her. "Maybe it's estrogen related," I suggested. She readily agreed to have blood tests done, and sure enough, her estrogen levels were practically nonexistent. But her reaction startled me. "Even though I can't do anything about it, at least now I know I'm not crazy," she said.

"What do you mean you can't do anything about it?" I asked.

"I can't take estrogen," she explained. "I have cystic breasts, and I've always been worried about breast cancer. How can I take a drug that may give me cancer?"

In spite of the growing evidence that hormone replacement

therapy is vital for many women's health, wellness, and longevity, only about 25 to 30 percent of menopausal women in the
United States are being treated with hormones. When I first
heard these numbers, I couldn't understand the reasoning. But
as I began to discuss women's reluctance to embark on this form
of therapy, one major fear kept coming up. Like my friend
Mary, many women are scared to death that estrogen replacement will give them cancer.

After doing serious research on this matter, and talking to
many experts, I believe that the estrogen-cancer connection has
been vastly overblown. Further, even some women who *do* have
a genetic risk of developing cancer may be better off taking estrogen. In many cases the good outweighs the bad. Rarely is this
position made public, or the real risks placed in the proper per-
spective. But I'm putting in my two cents' worth as a nonmed-
ical, self-educated woman who suffered terribly from the effects
of estrogen deprivation. I felt that I must address the estrogen-
cancer controversy in this book and try to alleviate some of the
fears.

## The Cancer Scare

In recent years there has been a massive scare campaign
launched by a lobby dedicated to breast cancer research, and almost violently opposed to hormone replacement therapy. This
lobby, led by Dr. Susan Love, a brilliant and dedicated breast
cancer surgeon, sees estrogen as an unreserved enemy. Her work
*Dr. Susan Love's Breast Book,* published in 1990, has been considered an invaluable resource on breast care and cancer pre-

vention. Recently Dr. Love has turned her attention to the controversy surrounding estrogen.

In *Dr. Susan Love's Breast Book,* she posits that estrogen poses unacceptable dangers for women. While readily acknowledging estrogen's role in significantly reducing the risks of heart disease and slowing the onset of both Alzheimer's disease and osteoporosis, Dr. Love insists that estrogen use is still unacceptably risky when the cancer rates are factored in.

As a breast cancer surgeon, Dr. Love has witnessed the horrors of that disease, and she is committed in her opposition to anything that might raise its risks. I can understand how easily a physician who deals with cancer every day can come to such a strong view, where *any* risk at all might seem too great. But I completely disagree with her position.

Many of her arguments come straight from the "menopause is not a disease" school of thinking. Why use a drug when there is no disease? As Love puts it, "When you talk about hormone replacement therapy for postmenopausal women, you're talking about women who have nothing wrong, who are normal, who may never get these diseases, and who are not necessarily at risk. There is no drug that is a free lunch. There are always side effects, so why would we put women on a drug that has the side effect of a potentially life-threatening disease?"

This is an interesting argument, especially coming from a doctor. The side effects of a drug do not always cancel out their greater good. We know, for instance, that aspirin can cause internal bleeding, but those with heart disease are advised to take one tablet each day; a headache may require two tablets. Beta blockers and calcium channel blockers given for heart disease have a number of deleterious side effects, as do all the cholesterol-lowering drugs. Still, the main effect is considered so vital as to mitigate the side effects. So it is with estrogen. Of course there are side effects, but in many instances a greater good has been served by the hormone's administration than by its reservation.

In a recent editorial piece in the *New York Times,* Dr. Love said, "Pharmaceutical companies defend their products by pointing out that one in three women die of heart disease, while only one in eight suffers from breast cancer. Although this is true, it is important to note that *in women younger than age seventy-five, there are three times as many deaths from breast cancer as there are from heart disease.*"

I am not a doctor, but I am an able researcher. I discovered that Dr. Love's statement is wrong. Her numbers are reversed. The facts are these. Women younger than age seventy-five die three times more often from heart disease than from breast cancer. In every age group, more women die of heart disease than of breast cancer. The mortality rate from heart disease as opposed to breast cancer soars as women grow older.

Furthermore, more than thirty scientific studies have attempted to find out if estrogen increases the breast cancer risk, and not one of them has shown a significant link. In spite of the controversy surrounding its use, scientists have yet to reach a definitive conclusion on estrogen. The National Institutes of Health, after evaluating more than thirty studies, said, "There is very little or no overall risk of breast cancer associated with the use of hormone replacement therapy." One recent study, published in the *Journal of the American Medical Association* (July 12, 1995), examined 1,000 women between the ages of fifty and sixty-four—about half of whom had earlier been diagnosed with breast cancer. The researchers "failed to find any increased risk of breast cancer associated with either current or long-term use of estrogen-progestin Hormone Replacement Therapy."

When I discussed the estrogen-cancer controversy with Dr. Klaiber, he presented an interesting hypothesis. "This debate about breast cancer and estrogen is not new," he told me. "In fact, there have been concerns about breast cancer for all of the fifty some years that estrogen replacement therapy has been available. Perhaps that, in itself, should be somewhat reassuring. If there really was a strong link between estrogen and breast cancer, it would have become readily apparent by now."

Dr. Klaiber is frustrated by how much of the antiestrogen rhetoric gives a false picture of the real risks of cancer versus the overwhelming benefits of estrogen. "I see women ten years into menopause who haven't taken estrogen because they are afraid of cancer," he said. "Meanwhile, their bones are thin and at risk of fracture, and their hearts may be at risk. When you consider that heart attacks are the leading cause of death in menopausal women, and kill five times as many women as breast cancer, you have to reevaluate."

Dr. Klaiber believes that the relationship between estrogen and breast cancer is not a strong one. "Look at the total picture," he urged. "Young women have the *lowest* incidence of breast cancer, but the *highest* levels of estrogen. On the other hand, older women have the *highest* incidence of breast cancer and the *lowest* levels of estrogen." Those facts should inform our thinking. We've always known that breast cancer increases dramatically with age, but we must ask, is the higher incidence of breast cancer in older women triggered by estrogen, or is it a by-product of living longer *because* of estrogen?

## The One-in-Nine Myth

What has women most alarmed is the frequent use of the "one-in-nine" figure to describe the risk of breast cancer. The figure implies that all women have a one-in-nine risk of developing the disease. But that's only true if you are eighty-five years old! The real risks for the majority of women aren't even close to that. For example, a fifty-year-old woman has only a one-in-*fifty* risk of developing breast cancer. And that assumes she has key risk factors.

Breast Cancer: The Risk by Age

| Age | Risk Factor |
|---|---|
| By 25 years | 1 in 19,608 |
| By 30 years | 1 in 2, 525 |
| By 40 years | 1 in 217 |
| By 50 years | 1 in 50 |
| By 60 years | 1 in 24 |
| By 70 years | 1 in 14 |
| By 80 years | 1 in 10 |
| By 85 years | 1 in 9 |

The risk of developing breast cancer is hardly negligible but also not inevitable. The risk is affected primarily by aging alone in the absence of other causative factors. Earlier detection, improved treatments, and continued research promise that the rates of breast cancer will continue to plummet. Rates have remained steady since the early 1980s.

Even these numbers still beg the question of whether *estrogen* is a factor in the risk. Here's one provocative question that received little airing: Is it possible that women undergoing hormone replacement therapy are living longer—and it is their greater longevity, not estrogen, that increases the cancer risk? Another way of posing the question might be: Are women choosing potentially longer life as a trade-off for the possible risk of cancer?

An analogy can be drawn with male prostate cancer. The statistics aren't very encouraging. In the last thirty-five years there has been a 17 percent increase in the incidence of prostate cancer. In the next year, more than 200,000 men will be diagnosed with prostate cancer, and some 35,000 will die from it. Pretty impressive figures. So impressive, in fact, that prostate cancer has almost pushed lung cancer off the top shelf of deadly killers.

Why is this happening? Is there an epidemic of prostate cancer? No. As with menopause, prostate cancer is one of the consequences of living longer. Breast cancer mostly afflicts older women, so you can say it is a consequence of our longer life spans as well.

## It's a Personal Choice

In the end, each woman must evaluate her own physiology and genetic predisposition versus the risks involved, and decide for herself which path she will follow. It is not the same for everyone. A woman with a high genetic risk of developing breast cancer may choose not to take estrogen—or to take it only for a limited time. However, the choice involves other considerations as well. She must evaluate her predisposition for other conditions. For example, is there a family history of heart disease? Did her grandmother or mother suffer from osteoarthritis? Is she small boned and light skinned—thus more susceptible to osteoporosis? Does she suffer from a thyroid condition? And finally, does she have a special sensitivity to estrogen deprivation? Is the *possible* added risk of breast cancer worth losing her quality of life, her sense of well-being, and perhaps her very sanity?

Julia found herself facing that decision when, without warning, her world unraveled. She thought she was going crazy, because there was no other explanation for why a healthy, happy forty-seven-year-old would suddenly snap. She was a therapist, and she could see no underlying cause. "My body was giving me signals, but I ignored them," she said, with a clarity refined over many years. "I had wonderful children, a great husband, intriguing work, a network of friends. It had to have been biochemical. But I couldn't recognize it." The litany of Julia's complaints was long: irregular periods, heavy bleeding, mood swings, crying jags, and sleeplessness. Then came her debilitating panic attacks. "It was around then that my husband's work took him out of town. I really began to have some terrible times. I was frightened. I felt helpless against the power of these feelings. But it was so radically out of character for me. I am a therapist, after all, and I couldn't make any sense out of it. My husband couldn't understand it either. He thought that perhaps I was manipulating him in an attempt to keep him at home. Of course, it really wasn't that at all. But I was in more trouble than he realized.

"When I finally had one of my panic attacks in the middle of town, and found myself unable to drive, I knew that I was going to have to take strong steps. I couldn't go on like this. I spoke with a colleague who does the same work I do, and it was she who first made the connection to menopause, and urged me to see a gynecologist. It was such a relief when she told me my estrogen levels were off. But I just couldn't handle the idea of estrogen replacement therapy. My best friend lost a breast to cancer, then another breast, and then it spread and she died. It was the most horrible thing I had ever witnessed. I asked my gynecologist if she could recommend an herbal estrogen treatment. She was the kind of doctor I could actually ask such a question of! Very up to date on homeopathic medicines. We had once discussed how many plants contained phytoestrogens and were natural sources of estrogen. But she burst my bubble. She said, 'These natural remedies are *still* estrogen.' I felt like crying. I needed help so desperately, but I felt the only help available might kill me. My doctor didn't treat me like a child. She was very straightforward. 'You're an intelligent woman,' she said. 'And right now you're responding to fear, not to facts. I'm going to give you some literature to read, and I want you also to talk this over with your husband.'

"I went home and read the data. I was somewhat surprised that the link between estrogen and cancer wasn't as solid as I had thought. Also, there was no breast cancer in my family history, and I didn't have other notable risks. Still, I couldn't get the picture of my friend out of my mind. My husband finally made the difference. He said, 'I'm going to be there for you, no matter what happens. You have to make the choice. But I know one thing, the way you're feeling now is real, and cancer is not. Can you live with this?' I realized, no, I couldn't. I asked my doctor to put me on estrogen."

As in so many other anecdotal reports of women in a state similar to Julia's, response to estrogen bordered on the miraculous. "Almost immediately after I began estrogen replacement therapy, I felt as if I had been reborn," she exclaimed. "It was as if I had stepped into the fountain of youth. I felt young, strong, and sexy. My fears vanished."

Anita is an example of what can happen when estrogen-sensitive women on hormone therapy discontinue estrogen for an indefinite period. She fell into a suicidal depression so deep that antidepressant medications proved worthless.

"I went off estrogen because I found a lump in my breast," Anita explained. "I had preliminary needle biopsies and was scheduled for more a few months later, so my gynecologist said, 'If you can stand it, why don't you try going off the estrogen?' So I figured I could stand it, and that's what I did. But by the end of two months, I was suicidal; I couldn't even get out of bed. It wasn't the blues. It was much worse than that. I can't even describe it.

"It started with catastrophic thinking. I felt that everything in my life was going to come to a terrible, crashing halt. It was the kind of thing where I'd take a fact, a true fact, like my husband's mother doesn't care for me, and extend it outward and end up with 'Everyone hates me. I've lost everything. I'm doomed.' That's how bad I felt. It was absolutely terrible."

"I went to a very good psychiatrist, and he put me on antidepressants. They didn't work. The subject of estrogen never came up with him. I didn't even think about it. Finally, when I was sitting in his office with him one day, he said, 'You know, I'm really stumped.' He couldn't understand why Zoloft, which is a very good antidepressant, wasn't having any effect. He said, 'I can't understand it. You haven't had any relief at all.' And I suddenly said to him, 'Oh, my God. Do you think this has anything to do with estrogen?' And he said, 'Well, it certainly could.' And we both sort of kicked ourselves for not having thought of this. But we didn't. I explained to him that I had gone off hormone therapy because of this lump in my breast.

"I called my oncologist and explained what had been going on. She immediately said, 'It sounds like you need estrogen. You'd better resume your estrogen replacement cycle and see if it helps. We'll keep a close eye on you, and if we have to change the dosage or take you off it again, we will.' I've only been back on estrogen for a few months now. I won't say that I'm completely better, but I'm not suicidal. I no longer feel my life is hopeless. I'm still on antidepressants, and now they're working better. But I *know* that without estrogen the antidepressants were meaningless."

I asked Anita if she was afraid. "I wonder how many women would have made the choice you did, thinking there was even the slightest possibility that estrogen could turn a precancerous lump into a cancerous condition."

"It's obviously a very personal decision," she replied. "But for me, it's the right one. I am confident that my doctors are carefully monitoring my condition. And meanwhile, while I was waiting for something that may never happen, I was losing everything that made my life worth living."

## The Progestin Conflict

When estrogen replacement was first prescribed in the 1960s, estrogen was used alone, not in combination with progestin. This was followed by a sharp increase in the number of women contracting endometrial cancer. It was discovered that unopposed estrogen taken over a period of ten or more years increased the risk of endometrial cancer four to ten times *more* than for women who didn't take the hormone—and the increased risk continued for up to fifteen years after cessation of estrogen therapy.

The reason is simple. Estrogen thickens the lining of the uterus. Before menopause, when a woman is still in her reproductive years, this thickening prepares the uterus for the fertilized egg. If an egg is not fertilized, the body produces progesterone, which causes the uterus to shed the lining in menstruation. Estrogen given after menopause also thickens the lining of the uterus, but without progesterone to trigger its shedding, the lining continues to build up. This can cause a precancerous condition called endometrial hyperplasia, and for some women it can lead to cancer.

Today the standard course of hormone replacement therapy for a woman with an intact uterus is a combination of estrogen and progestin, usually taken cyclically. This offers protection against endometrial cancer. However, as was demonstrated in my case, it's somewhat more complex than that.

For many women, the addition of progestin creates symptoms that range from uncomfortable to unacceptable. In fact, statistics show that the number-one reason women stop hormone replacement altogether is that they cannot cope with the return of monthly periods—an effect of progestin. Progestin can cause PMS-like symptoms, including severe depression, for women who are susceptible.

So what is a woman in these circumstances to do? The first step is to have her doctor experiment with dosage and combination levels. In severe cases, a doctor may recommend unopposed estrogen with the caveat that a woman receive annual endometrial biopsies to check the thickness of the uterine lining. If her lining thickens beyond acceptable levels, the doctor can then prescribe short-term progestin.

A continuous combined regimen of estrogen and progestin will eliminate monthly bleeding, but even a very low dose of progestin taken daily will be difficult for women who react strongly to the hormone.

## New Advances

Fortunately, hormone replacement therapy is a work in progress. Researchers continue to design different combinations and delivery systems that will solve these problems. A new patch, recently made available, delivers very low doses of both estrogen and progestin. Because the patch technology is so effective, doses of both hormones can be delivered which achieve optimal results—without the side effects. Also, a natural progesterone gel will soon be available for menopausal women. This gel can be concentrated in the uterus, rather than in the blood, eliminating side effects.

Scientists are also testing the addition of small amounts of the male hormone testosterone to the therapy. According to Dr. Elizabeth Barrett-Conner, a world renowned researcher at the University of California, San Diego, School of Medicine, "For some women, it appears as if androgen is the missing hormone of the perimenopausal years. They can feel depressed, fatigued and, particularly, experience a loss of libido, or sex drive—all of which respond to androgen therapy." While this research is ongoing, it presents yet another avenue of potential help for women suffering from hormone imbalances.

Researchers have also been working on the next generation of hormone replacement therapy drugs. These are compounds called SERMS, or Selective Estrogen Receptor Modulators. SERMS were discovered when researchers studied the effects of tamoxifen on women with breast cancer. It had previously been assumed that women had one specific kind of estrogen receptor—when the hormone was present, the entire body would react. Tamoxifen was supposed to shut down those receptors, the theory being that starving the receptors would help prevent or shrink tumors in breast cancer patients. However, it was accepted theory that if estrogen were denied to one part of the body, it would also be depleted elsewhere. But researchers discovered that while tamoxifen did *deny estrogen* to receptors in the breast tissue, it *behaved as estrogen* in the bones. This led them to theorize that perhaps estrogen was more selective than they had previously believed. It didn't have the same effect on every cell. They then constructed more selective artificial hormones.

Researchers are investigating the possibility that there are many different kinds of estrogen receptors, and that their response can be controlled by a SERM that is delivered to the specific site. By chance, tamoxifen proved to shrink breast tumors and protect the bones, but raised the risk of uterine cancer. There are now a generation of SERMs ready to be launched; these will behave as estrogen in both the bones and the heart, while protecting the breasts and the uterus from any increased risk of exposure.

The missing element is still the brain—which has a controlling influence on all bodily systems, and receives messages from neurotransmitters. But the possibility exists that in the future scientists will develop a form of estrogen replacement therapy that will allow women to tailor their treatments to receive all of the benefits and none of the negative side effects.

I find it curious that Dr. Susan Love responds to the possibility of new research discoveries with cynicism. Recently, she said, "Scientists are hoping to use some of this new information to design the perfect hormone: one that will protect the uterus and breast from cancer, stop hot flashes, and prevent osteoporosis and heart disease. It would be lovely—could it do housework too?—but I'm skeptical. It would still be a drug. And I have yet to see a drug that doesn't have some side effects."

I believe we can never close the door on our future. What if we had done that before the development of estrogen replacement therapy?

The failure of women to recognize the risks of menopause is of great concern to Dr. Klaiber. "As a result of that failure, many women who should benefit from estrogen are not doing so." He acknowledges that women are concerned about uterine and breast cancer. "My experience at a meeting of the North American Menopause Society emphasized this in a way that surprised me," he told me. "When the issue of uterine cancer came up, one of the women said that she felt that women had been lied to in the 1960s and 1970s about the safety of estrogen. I do not think that was the case. It was primarily a lack of information on the part of the medical profession regarding the necessity to prescribe progestins with estrogen. Unfortunately, the legacy of that time still exists. The present data strongly support that the progestins protect against uterine cancer and that any increased risk of breast cancer associated with estrogen administration is quite small and greatly outweighed by the benefits achieved in the areas of cardiovascular disease and osteoporosis. It is vital that women understand the importance of estrogen to their health."

Estrogen saved my life. Estrogen saved my sanity. Knowing that I can protect my heart and fight the effects of osteoporosis as well is an added bonus. I feel confident that with regular checkups, including mammograms and gynecological examinations, I have more than a fighting chance of early detection and treatment of any cancer that might develop. I am very much in the *pro* estrogen camp. I am interested in the quality of life as well as in it quantity. I believe that my continued use of estrogen provides me with the best chance for both.

# 10

# Listen to Your Body

There was a time, not all that long ago, before the proliferation of medical experts, clinical trials, and specialists who treated every malady, when women had no choice but to do what was natural. They listened to their bodies. They trusted their experience, and that of their mothers and grandmothers before them. Although we now live in an exciting era with increasingly sophisticated means of diagnosis and treatment, many of our scientific and medical advances have created further barriers between patient and doctor. People often feel as if they have no role in their own diagnosis. How often does a physician ask a patient her opinion? So many patients accept at face value whatever their doctors tell them, even when it negates their own experience. If they say, "I have a problem," and their doctors tell them, "No, you don't," they are more inclined to believe the doctors than they are themselves!

Women are especially vulnerable to having their symptoms dismissed by doctors. The failure on the physician's part may have less to do with a lack of knowledge than with the fact that the patient is a woman. Gender bias is still widespread in medicine—you even see it displayed by female doctors. They were trained in the same atmosphere as men, and so adopt many of the same unconscious attitudes.

Although most women in their forties and fifties are healthy, vital, sexually active, and engaged fully in life, they are still haunted by outdated attitudes about menopause. A woman of fifty who complains to her doctor about depression, anxiety, panic attacks, or other nonspecific problems can more often than not expect the physician initially to judge them to be emotional rather than physical problems. As recently as 1987, a textbook discussing menopause warned doctors: "Emotional instability is an outstanding feature of this phase of life. Nervousness and anxiety are extremely frequent. The patient may feel that the end of her useful life has come, that now she is old, that she has lost her appeal as a woman, and that nothing is left to her. She cries easily; she flares up at her family and friends; she is irritable and may have difficulty in composing her thoughts or her reactions."

Believe it or not, this view is privately held by a large number of doctors. Women have described to me how their gynecologists or internists regarded them with pity when they described their symptoms, as if to say, "I know it's hard for you to get older." Marilyn, a gorgeous, fifty-two-year-old actress, said her doctor completely ignored her physical complaints. "He just stared at me with this funny smile, and then he said, 'When a woman is as beautiful as you are, it can be very traumatic to see that beauty fading.' I was outraged. I snapped at him, 'I didn't come here to have my looks analyzed. I came here to get a damn blood test!'"

Janice, a successful, happy, and well-balanced forty-eight-year-old business woman, was not the least bit worried about the approach of menopause. "I was secure in myself," she said. She was not prepared, however, for the eruption of physical and emotional symptoms. She suddenly fell into a deep depression for no apparent reason. Her periods became so horrible that she couldn't leave her apartment. "I knew there was a physical reason for this," she said. "I went to my gynecologist, and I said, 'Look, I'm not an alarmist, I'm not a crybaby. I'm a rational person, but I don't feel very rational right now. Something is happening to my body. I've never experienced anything like this before, and, frankly, I'm very worried. I'm afraid I may have cancer or something.'

"I was expecting him to offer me a medical diagnosis," Janice continued. "Instead, he shrugged and replied matter-of-factly, 'You've never been this age before.' I felt as though he hadn't heard a word I'd said. Never been this age before? Now what was *that* supposed to mean? He told me that many women get depressed and have some heavy periods before menopause, and it should pass. He also suggested that I see a therapist. And that was it. He didn't even bother to examine me. Nothing. I was shaking with rage by the time I left the office. He actually believed that my age explained away the reasons for my symptoms!"

Janice was hearing a response that is all too common when women seek help from doctors. The gender bias in treatment has been documented. In one study, John McKinlay, M.D., videotaped visits to doctor's offices made by patients matched for every variable but gender. The films showed that a man and a woman who complained of the same symptoms were often treated very differently. Men were twice as likely to be referred to a medical specialist, and women were much likelier to be referred to a psychotherapist. Dr. McKinlay concluded that the gender-related disparities apparent in much medical literature may reflect what doctors see rather than actual physiological disorders. These results give us further reason to be concerned. Even though a manifest number of symptoms occur in the perimenopause, what a woman relates is what she experiences. There is nothing for a physician to see.

Another survey of 253 primary care physicians concluded, "Among physicians' attitudes about women, the most frequently mentioned are the beliefs that women are more emotionally unstable and volatile than men, apt to internalize emotional upsets as physical problems, and consequently likely to have a higher prevalence of psychosomatic illness than men do."

This is particularly true if a doctor can pinpoint an external event as the "cause" of symptoms. Ruth is a case in point. She was overwhelmed by the ferocity of her symptoms. "There were mood changes, irregular cycles, and pain," Ruth said. "First I started having really bad pain with my period. Then I'd get depressed, and I became prone to these mood swings. I got really nasty, too. I didn't want to do anything. I was terrible to people, just terrible. I started bleeding very heavily sometimes during my period, and the rest of the time I had sort of a bloated heaviness low in my pelvis. There was just no relief. And to top it off, my insomnia kept getting worse and worse. Everyone, including my doctor, blamed it on nerves. I had just gotten a divorce. I'm aware that going through a divorce is stressful. But I knew this wasn't about the divorce, and nobody would listen. I finally had to go to a different doctor. I didn't even *mention* the divorce. Only then was I able to get some medical help." Ruth's doctor found that her estrogen levels were severely depleted. She prescribed hormone replacement therapy, and Ruth's symptoms disappeared almost overnight.

Margie received the same reaction from her family and friends when she complained of excessive fatigue and an upheaval in her feelings. Margie had always had a very quiet temperament, but her moods began sending her into spontaneous rages at one moment and fits of crying at the next. Since her last child had recently left home to go to college in another state, her doctor was amused that she hadn't figured it out. "Haven't you ever heard of the empty nest syndrome?" he asked, sure of his diagnosis. Margie left his office feeling thoroughly misunderstood, and with a few sample packets of the antianxiety drug lorazepam in her purse.

It's difficult to convey the agony of crying out for help and being summarily dismissed. One woman described it this way: "It's like one of those slow-motion nightmares, where you're in danger and you're trying to scream so someone nearby will see you, and nothing comes out of your mouth. You wake up in a cold sweat, with your heart pounding."

"Part of the problem," says Dr. Klaiber bluntly, "is that the American medical profession is mainly men." But it's not only the male physicians. "Women physicians aren't necessarily more understanding because they are women," declares Dr.

Elizabeth Vliet in her book *Screaming to Be Heard*. "All physicians have been taught by the same flawed system of education that does not fully *hear* women's voices, does not adequately address women's body differences or value women's insights and women's experiences. Women physicians have been taught the same negative stereotypes of female patients as have male doctors."

Sadly, too many women respond by trying to hide their symptoms. "Most women know their bodies so well that I think they intuitively feel a hormonal connection," said Margaret, a social worker in private practice. "They're just reluctant to talk about it." Margaret thinks she knows why. "We're afraid to mention what's going on because people might think we're going crazy."

"One of the problems," Margaret added, "is that doctors don't test hormone levels automatically, the way you have a breast exam every two years or a Pap smear every year. But they should. I know my body so well that several times over the years I've called my doctor and said, 'I don't have enough estrogen.' And she would ask me, 'How do you know?' And I would answer, 'Because I know. She'd indulge me—that's what it felt like, an *indulgence*—and she'd check my hormone levels. Sure enough, every time, the tests came back showing low estrogen levels."

Margaret remained astonished that her doctor was so unreceptive. "Can you believe it?" she asked. "My doctor's a woman and she doesn't believe me! I'm trying to educate *her*, and she just looks at me. At one point, when I said that I was going to take natural testosterone, she asked, 'How are you going to do that?' I said, 'They put it in a uterine cream and you rub it on your genitals.' She just stared at me like I was a witch!"

The menopausal transition is a challenging time, and it shakes the confidence of many women. There's quite a lot for a woman to deal with as she makes her way through the medical system. But even when a woman intuitively knows or is educated to know that there are biological reasons for her terrifying panic attacks or debilitating depression, there is often a resistance to getting professional help.

"As a therapist, I see women in my practice who have symptoms that are clearly hormonally related," says Elizabeth. "So I ask them to go back to their doctors for tests. Some are reluctant to do that. In fact, I had one client who left treatment because I told her she needed a new doctor. She clearly had a hormonal problem, and her doctor just wouldn't do the tests for her. She had all the symptoms—the depression, the anxiety, the hot flashes, everything. But she just couldn't stand up to this male authority figure."

"We need to educate physicians," says Karen, a psychiatrist who found herself in a delicate situation with her own gynecologist. Not only was he a colleague but his office was only a few doors down from her own. "He's an 'I know best' doctor," she said wryly. "But as it turns out, he doesn't know best. I'm a blue-eyed blonde with a grandmother who had a hump, and I never liked milk. I've always known I had a risk of osteoporosis, and I figured I was a good candidate for estrogen therapy. So as soon as my periods started becoming the least bit irregular, I asked him about hormone replacement. He said, 'I don't believe in it.' I never said a word, but I decided I had to find another doctor. When I called his office to have my records transferred, his administrative assistant said, 'But why? You've been his patient for a long time.' I told her that he wouldn't even have a discussion with me about estrogen replacement. I explained that I'd been reading the literature, educating myself, and I was convinced it was right for me. I told her, 'If he doesn't believe in it, I don't think he's keeping up with things.'" Karen's experience is an object lesson for everyone. "If we don't educate each other," she said, "nobody else is going to do it."

New York University clinical professor of psychology, Dr. Marcia Levy-Warren, whose skills allow her special insight into the connection between biology and the brain, told me about her experience.

"In a relatively short period of time, I saw five different women who were between the ages of forty-two and forty-seven," she said. "One was a personal friend of mine, and four were patients. All of them seemed to be in pretty good psychological health, but they were having symptoms of what they referred to as 'anxiety.' All of them basically described symptoms such as heart palpitations. They also complained of suddenly getting very hot, and feeling unusually moody and volatile. Then they'd feel panicked by how they were feeling physically, and their symptoms would escalate."

Fearful that they were having heart problems, the women went to their internists. Some were referred to psychiatrists, who put them on Prozac, and others were put on Prozac by their internists. But Prozac didn't relieve the symptoms, and by the time they consulted Dr. Levy-Warren, they felt worse than ever.

"It's true that each of these women had a particular problem with separation, or feelings of abandonment," Dr. Levy-Warren observed. "All of them had issues about the impending end of their childbearing years; two of them had never had children and were feeling very conflicted. They were entertaining notions about still trying to have a baby. Still, I felt that this was not a purely psychiatric problem. It seemed to me that there was a biological connection to the psychological manifestations."

One of Dr. Levy-Warren's standard diagnostic tools was to ask each woman about the major physiological events in her life—such as when she got her first period or when she experienced growth spurts. She understood that these events had a psychological relevance.

"In the course of these discussions, I would ask, 'Are you having any perimenopausal or menopausal symptoms?' and I discovered that all of them had irregular periods. The overall scenario was that their periods were different than they used to be—they lasted a shorter time, were often more intense, and were more frequent."

In each case, Dr. Levy-Warren told me, the woman experienced a jolt of awareness—like a lightbulb going on—that there was a rhythm to her emotional symptoms. That rhythm was related to her cycles. Dr. Levy-Warren was able to conclude that the bursts of hormonal activity triggered the emotional responses.

As I review what happened to me, I cannot help wondering: Could I have avoided my personal "madness," the hell into which I descended alone and unknowing, had someone like Dr. Levy-Warren been a part of my medical life at the time?

## What Every Woman Can Do

Albert Camus wrote that "the evolution of the body, like that of the mind, has its history, its reversals, its gains, and its losses." Each of us experiences the truth of this as we pass from one stage of life to another. And it is the *unique* history of each woman's body that sets the standard for that woman's treatment. This is why it is so critical that doctors study the individual, not just the malady.

I look forward to a time when every physician is fully educated, aware, and in tune with the necessary therapy to treat women's hormonal changes. In the meantime, however, it is up to us—the women who are *living* these changes—to hold our physicians accountable, and to arm ourselves with knowledge.

It is the gradual, almost imperceptible shift in the hormonal balance in the perimenopause to which women need to be alerted. By the time the symptom-producing threshold has been crossed, a woman may already be experiencing severe physical and psychological changes. In these cases, perimenopause is like a thief in the night. The best way to avoid being robbed of well-being is to be prepared. Every woman can do this by having a blood test around age forty (or before, if there is a history of hormonal imbalance, or there has been a hysterectomy) to establish a *baseline* for estrogen levels. Along with that, women should establish a baseline for symptoms so they can easily detect any changes. Some women even keep charts of their cycles and symptoms throughout adulthood, as a regular part of their health records.

Since the onset of menopause, with its gradual depletion of

estrogen, is impossible to pinpoint, and since the range of symptoms is so vast and disparate, if a woman were to have a baseline estrogen evaluation, then when she began to sense changes in her mood or disquieting physical symptoms, it would be relatively simple to do some comparative testing to determine whether her symptoms reflected a significant decrease in the production of estrogen.

Dr. Ari Birkenfeld, associate professor of reproductive endocrinology at Mt. Sinai Hospital in New York, suggests an even more comprehensive approach. "Since estrogen doesn't maintain a steady level, and one cycle is not necessarily like the next one, you would have to first take a look at a woman's entire profile," he says. "You wouldn't just look at estrogen. There are both clinical and endocrine signs you can evaluate. For instance, shortening of the cycle is one sign. You can do a test of estrogen and FSH production. And you can do a challenge test of the ovaries, which involves giving a woman the drug Clomid. Clomid will show if there is an exaggerated increase in FSH, and then you can tell if there is a decline in the ovaries."

Dr. Edward Klaiber notes there are other factors that may need consideration as well. "In the depressed women we studied, we found that many of their estrogen levels were fine," he said. "But for some reason, their bodies weren't clearing it. So if you only look at estrogen levels, you may not see the entire picture." He suggested that women who experience all of the symptoms yet show no real decline in estrogen should ask to have other hormone levels evaluated. In his study group, Klaiber tested metabolic production and clearance rate. It's a complicated measure in which radioactive tracer amounts of both estrogen and testosterone are given; these allow a doctor to determine how much of each hormone the body is producing.

"We found that these women had a testosterone abnormality," Dr. Klaiber said. "Testosterone was being produced at three times its normal level, while at the same time there was a reduced metabolic clearance of estrogen. Since testosterone is an antiestrogen, we realized that these depressed women had a very marked production of antiestrogen, which was interfering with the estrogen receptors. If you don't have a sufficient estrogen effect, the receptors will begin to atrophy. Even though these women had sufficient estrogen production, their bodies couldn't metabolize the estrogen normally. We gave them extremely high doses of estrogen in an attempt to prime their estrogen receptors. It worked."

The implications of this study are staggering, not only for severely depressed menopausal women but for severely depressed *non*menopausal women. What physician would ever think of checking a young, depressed woman's testosterone level as a possible cause of her depression? Probably none. For these women the psychiatrist's office, with a prescription for antidepressants or antipsychotics, is the therapy of choice.

Individuality is the key to treatment. As long as doctors are looking at broad diagnostic standards, it's likely that women will continue to fall through the cracks. Dr. Bruce McEwen feels very strongly about this. "Women need to realize that there are tremendous individual differences in biology that we don't completely understand," he said. "They may have to do with internal states of neurochemistry that make the brains in some people more susceptible to psychological illness than others— even when they have the same hormone levels. But they're not

crazy; it's really happening! The problem is that the medical profession tends to work with norms. If someone is off the scale,
that person doesn't get attended to."

Even if only 10 or 15 percent of the 70 million women who
are about to enter menopause end up with a psychiatric disorder, that is still as many as 10.5 million women. The tragedy is
compounded by the fact that a majority of those women have
families, husbands, children, friends, and colleagues—all of
whose lives may be needlessly affected. If that's "off the scale,"
perhaps it's time that doctors used a different scale!

## The Therapy Connection

For some women, like myself, hormonal chaos in the
perimenopause affects the brain as if it were a symphony or-
chestra where each section is playing to its own tune and
rhythm. The result is a cacophony of sound, an assault on the
senses. While this is an experience replicated by many women
in the menopausal years, every woman's transition is unique.
There are complex genetic patterns that are as individual as fin-
gerprints; no two sets are identical. Each woman's reaction to
the alteration in hormones that occurs during any of the major
female transition periods is influenced by a number of factors:
her age, her history, her life situation at the time, her feelings
and perceptions, and so on. That lays the groundwork for a lot
of variation in behavior. Yet for most women who experience
the loss of a sense of well-being or depression, estrogen replacement is the miraculous restorer.

There is, however, a second element. For women like myself
who have been wrenched from desperate, terrifying, often per-

ilous circumstances, whose perimenopausal transitions have been disabling experiences, therapeutic intervention is an important catalyst for repairing and reintegrating a fragmented self.

If estrogen replacement to correct my hormonal imbalance was the featured player in bringing about my recovery, the psychoanalytic situation was the dramatic setting; it was both text and context. Therapy is a kind of psychological hothouse where quiet miracles of transformation take place. It is where I came to understand the effects of estrogen loss as a contributing factor in feelings of confusion and dislocation, and to separate out the physical factors from the psychological ones.

More than that, I came to see therapy as a *physical* treatment—as closely linked to the neuropathways as estrogen itself. And my experience was validated by experts. Dr. McEwen affirmed for me that trauma actually causes structural changes in the brain by altering the brain's circuitry. Dr. Michael Jenike, director of the Clinic for Treatment of Obsessive-Compulsive Disorders at the Massachusetts General Hospital, impressed upon me that behavioral treatments can have biological effects. "Psychotherapy can produce changes in brain function similar to those seen with psychiatric medicine," he emphasized. Thus, the prolonged stress from clinical depression or the severe abuse to the brain from an acute psychotic episode begs for psychotherapeutic intervention. Estrogen treatment alone may not be able to restore the confidence and self-esteem that have been so badly damaged.

Lynn discovered that lesson. Today, she is an energetic, fit, and lovely fifty-eight-year-old woman who runs a fashionable boutique. But just a few years ago she wouldn't have believed that such a transformation was in the realm of possibility. Lynn had an easy transition into menopause in her early fifties, and by the time she was fifty-three she didn't even think about menopause anymore. "I thought I was living proof of the new woman, who barely blinked at menopause," she told me, laughing. "I'd never felt better." Then one morning she woke up and couldn't stand the idea of leaving the house. "I had a big meeting planned with a buyer, and I couldn't face it," she said. "I didn't know why, but it filled me with dread. It was like a very strong psychic message that it was dangerous for me to leave my house. For the next week, I was a basket case. I felt jittery, tingly, scared for no reason. It felt like I was having a nervous breakdown. Finally, I called my doctor, and he referred me to a psychiatrist."

For a solid year, Lynn dragged herself to the psychiatrist's office three times a week. "During each session, we would take this long, convoluted journey back to my childhood," she said ruefully. "Sometimes he would use hypnosis. Even though I had wonderful parents and a happy childhood, and had always been a very balanced and confident person, this doctor convinced me that I was suffering from childhood traumas which destroyed my self-esteem. The longer I went to him, the more I felt like a worm. I didn't know who I was anymore, and my phobias were getting worse. I was afraid to leave the house. I stopped seeing almost everyone except my psychiatrist. He dominated my life completely."

Ultimately, Lynn was rescued from this nightmare by a routine visit to her gynecologist. "He told me he wanted to put me on estrogen replacement therapy, because it would protect my bones and heart. I said okay, but I didn't give it much thought. Then, about a week after I started, I woke up one morning and my head was clear. I actually felt good. And the feeling lasted. What really convinced me I was better was that I didn't want to keep my psychiatrist appointment. Somehow I sensed it would spoil this wonderful way I was feeling."

With new clarity, Lynn saw that her symptoms had been physical, not mental. She quit her psychiatrist. However, in the aftermath of a year's trauma, she felt deflated, humiliated, less than she had been. "I was better," she said, "but I was sad, too. I felt as if I'd never completely recover the 'me' I had lost. When a friend suggested I go see her therapist, I didn't expect much. But this woman opened my eyes. She became my ally. Over the years she has led me back, painstakingly, to the self I once was. Without her, estrogen would have been only a partial solution."

Psychotherapy can be a vital adjunct to hormone replacement for women like Lynn and myself whose circuits have been affected by going so long without treatment. Furthermore, for any woman who has suffered through a long period of mental illness caused by hormonal imbalance, therapy can help gain an understanding of her experience in a setting that is sympathetic and nonjudgmental.

## A Final Thought

My own experience proved to me that there is nothing predictable about menopause except menopause itself. My own menopause's beginnings were stealthy and insidious. There was no sudden flash, none of the known predictables. If I had been capable of recognizing and connecting my symptoms to declining estrogen levels, or had my problem been routinely discovered during clinical testing, I might have been spared a harrowing ordeal. But that was not to be. I'd like to think this book may help other women avoid my experience.

Most discussions relating to midlife present it as a time of freedom and liberation, as an opportunity for spiritual growth, for self-transformation and self-transcendence. Midlife issues revolve around how women define themselves and the challenges that await them. But for some of us these ideas have no meaning. When our hormone levels destabilize, our brains become compromised, and we become emotionally trapped. If we are helpless before our biology, how are we liberated? If we cannot transcend our physical selves, how do we move beyond the immediacy of our lives to grasp its spiritual dimension?

It has nothing to do with one's "will" or one's ability to "tough it out." The evidence is overwhelming. Women who suffer a psychological disorder during any of the major female transitions are genetically prone to develop this condition. The dramatic therapeutic response to hormone replacement premenstrually, postpartumly, and menopausally goes far to support that notion that these psychological disorders are organic and biologically triggered.

Is biology destiny? There are women who are susceptible to mental illness. Can all of their problems be solved with hormone replacement therapy? No, of course not. But as scientists continue to chart the complex genetic patterns that account for predispositions to certain diseases and illnesses, more and more information is being collected every day. That information will help doctors make more informed choices, and will generate research into drugs and compounds that will someday treat a wide range of hormone-related maladies.

Does our biology have to be our destiny? If we intend to preserve the quality of our lives, we have to educate ourselves. The women whose personal struggles fill these pages have helped us do that. They have highlighted some of the frustrating realities that women face. They have made us more aware of the walls of ignorance we come up against, again and again, when we turn to our own physicians for help. If there is any message in the recounting of these tragic stories, it is this. A woman needs to learn everything she can about her changing hormones. Then, fortified with that information, she must insist that every medical test she needs be done.

If women refuse to do this, we will hasten not only our physical death but the death of our creative, feeling, spiritually transcendent selves. We will have wasted—tragically sacrificed—the most liberating and deeply fulfilling years of our lives.

# Afterword:

# The Meeting of Biology and Psychotherapy

Ralph Wharton, M.D.

Clinical Professor of Psychiatry,
Columbia University College of Physicians and Surgeons

There has been an intuitive knowledge of the role of hormones as far back as the famous *castrati*. It was understood that the ability to sing high notes demanded by the Church's most sacred music was best preserved by the castration of its finest young singers. Eunuchs, who guarded the harems of sultans and emperors, also paid a high hormonal price, but they often accrued great power.

It wasn't until the 1930s, however, that a more specific and therapeutic understanding of the thyroid, pituitary, and male and female sex hormones came to light. That understanding is still evolving. Even today many mysteries surround the hormonal system. There are endless questions still unanswered about hormonal relations to the mind-body continuum—especially concerning our adaptations to certain stress and sex hormones. Both the body and the mind are powerfully affected by the varying levels of hormones circulating throughout.

It has only recently been found that there are two kinds of receptor sites for estrogen in the female body. It is a given that estrogen plays a powerful role in the reproductive system, but its effects are far more widespread than previously believed. In men, levels of estrogen may affect the function of the prostate gland as well as bone density. In menopausal women, sensitivity to declining estrogen levels can vary from overt psychosis or mild depression to no discernible change in mood or function. In other words, the personal variables are enormous. The true effects of estrogen on mood are just beginning to be more fully researched. It is possible that a small regulating dose of estrogen will allow many women to forgo the use of antianxiety or antidepressant medications altogether.

Marcia Lawrence is an unusually sensitive and talented writer who has given us a view of the delusional world in which she suffered from hearing voices and developing magical beliefs. Concomitantly, she experienced a gradual and inexorable decline in estrogen hormone production. Both inner (bodily) and outer (sensory) sensitivities contributed to her disturbance in cognition and mood.

While I am thoroughly familiar with the role of estrogen in mental activity, there was a substantial delay in her receiving hormone therapy. The delay, in retrospect, came in part because the gynecologist who referred her to me had found no disturbance during his examination. It was only after some months of treatment that her flood of feelings and bodily sensations suggested a hormonal disorder. Ultimately, I did order blood tests, which confirmed the situation.

Menopausal symptoms had evolved uniquely during the course of Marcia's psychotherapy in a most striking manner. The "special" logic of her nightmare unraveled. In one of her early dreams, she announced, "I am writing a book and the title is 'Emergence and Identity.'" Unwittingly, or perhaps intuitively, she felt she was emerging from her prolonged grief reaction and developing a different identity—that of a writer whose talent surfaced in and gave expression to menopause. Her individual intense psychotherapy was an invaluable support early on, before the diagnosis was clear. Her capacity for trust, dreamwork, and insight helped stabilize her mood before any significant hormonal treatment.

It is impossible to be precise about the set point of sensitivity for hormonal awareness. For despite generally positive feelings there were moments of flooding which suggested a hormonal tide change in this sensitive woman. I ordered the appropriate blood tests, and hormonal levels were obtained. The subsequent prescription for medication provided further ample positive response to treatment. There is no question that the medication promoted treatment response. It is highly likely that an earlier determination and the earlier prescription of hormone replacement would have speeded improvement in her interpersonal issues and the resolution of her loss.

While it is unlikely that all mental mechanisms would become unhinged in this way, it is likely that a cascade of chemical events were precipitated by gradual estrogen deprivation. What is clear is that estrogen had dramatic benefits for Marcia—and that as a therapeutic tool it has definitely been underutilized.

Others will benefit from wider use of this hormone in menopausal and perimenopausal depression. Marcia Lawrence's own vivid experience clarifies this beyond question.

# Bibliography

Angier, Natalie. "New Respect for Estrogen's Influence." *New York Times,* June 24, 1997.

Baron Faust, Rita. "Welcome to Perimenopause: Life in Hormonal Limbo." *American Health,* January–February 1995.

Berlin, Fred S., M.D., Ph.D. et al. "Periodic Psychosis of Puberty: A Case Report." *Am. J. Psychiatry,* January 1982, 139:1.

Brisco, Paula, and Karla Morales. *The Hormone Replacement Handbook.* People's Medical Society, 1996.

Brody, Jane E. "Alzheimer Studies Thwarted: Women Convinced of Benefits Do Not Want Placebo." *New York Times,* March 5, 1997.

———."Drug Researchers Working to Design Customized Estrogen." *New York Times,* March 4, 1997.

———."Estrogen After Menopause? A Tough Dilemma." *New York Times,* August 20, 1997.

Endo, M. Daiguji, et al. "Peridoic Psychosis Recurring in Association with Menstrual Cycle." *Journal of Clinical Psychiatry,* 1978, 39.

Gallagher, Winifred, "Midlife Myths." *Atlantic Monthly,* May 1993.

Gilbert, Susan. "Estrogen Patch Appears to Lift Severe Depression in New Mothers." *New York Times,* May 1, 1996.

Gladwell, Malcolm. "The Estrogen Question: How Wrong Is Susan Love?" *New Yorker,* June 9, 1997.

Glover, Vivette, and Peter Liddle, et al. "Mild Hypomania (the Highs) Can Be a Feature of the First Postpartum Week Associated with Later Depression." *British Journal of Psychiatry*, 1994, 164.

Hamilton, James Alexander, and Patricia Neel Harberger. *Postpartum Psychiatric Illness*. University of Pennsylvania Press, Philadelphia, Pa., 1992.

Handley, S.L., T.L. Dunn, J.M. Baker, et al. "Mood Changes in the Puerperium and Plasma Tryptophan and Cortisol Concentrations. *British Medical Journal*, 1977.

Hay, Alistair G., et al. "Affective Symptoms in Women Attending a Menopause Clinic." *British Journal of Psychiatry*, 1994, 164:513–16.

Henderson, Victor W., M.D. "Alzheimer's Disease in Women: Is There a Role for Estrogen Replacement Therapy?" *Menopause Management*, vol. 4, no. 6 (1995).

Hoffman, Eileen, M.D. *Our Health, Our Lives: A Revolutionary Approach to Total Health Care for Women*. New York: Pocket Books, 1995.

Klaiber, Edward, M.D., et al. "Estrogen Therapy for Severe Persistent Depressions in Women." *Archives of General Psychiatry*, May 1979, vol. 36.

Kotulak, Ronald. *Inside the Brain: Revolutionary Discoveries of How the Mind Works*. Kansas City, MO: Andrews McMeel Publishing, 1996. P. 126.

Landsberg Warga, Claire. "Estrogen and the Brain." *New York*, August 11, 1997.

Levy-Warren, Marcia, Ph.D. *The Adolescent Journey*. Northvale, N.J.: Jason Aronson, Inc., 1996.

Luine, Victoria N., Cheryl F. Harding, editors. *Hormonal Restructuring of the Adult Brain*. New York Academy of Sciences, New York, 1994, vol. 743.

Maes, M. et al. "Hypothalmic-Pituitary-Adrenal and -Thyroid Axis Dysfunctions and Decrements in the Availability of L-Tryptophan as Biological Markers of Suicidal Ideation in Major Depressed Females." *Acta Psychiatr. Scan.*, 1989,80:13–17

Mann, John J., M.D., and Sititij Kapur, M.D. "The Emergence of Suicidal Ideation and Behavior During Antidepressant Pharmacotherapy." *Arch. Gen. Psychiatry*, vol 48, 1991.

Nash, Madeleine. "Early Flash Points." *Time*, April 21, 1997.

———."Every Woman's Dilemma." *Time*, June 30, 1997.

Okasha, A., et al. "Panic Disorder an Overlapping or Independent Entity?" *British Journal of Psychiatry*, 1994, 164:818–25.

Parker, Gordon, et.al. "Defining Melancholia: Properties of a Refined Sign-Based Measure," *British Journal of Psychiatry*, 1994, 164.

Pecins-Thompson, M., N.A. Barown, C.L. Bethea, "Regulation of Serotonin Reuptake Transporter (SERT) mRNA Expression by Estrogen (E) and Progesterone (P) in Rhesus Macaques, Abstract #571.5, Annual Meeting of The Society for Neuroscience, 1996.

Rako, Susan, M.D. *The Hormone of Desire: The Truth About Sexuality, Menopause, and Testosterone.* New York: Harmony Books, 1995.

Restak, Richard M., M.D. *Receptors.* New York: Bantam Books, 1994.

Rockmore, Abigail L., and Stone Phillips. "New Mother's Nightmare." *20/20*, ABC News, August 2, 1991.

Schmidt, Peter J., M.D., and David R. Rubinow, M.D. "Menopause Related Affective Disorders: A Justification for Further Study." *Amer. Journal Psychiatry*, 1991, 149:844–52.

Scully, James H., ed. *Psychiatry.* Baltimore, MD: Williams and Wilkins, 1996.

Shapiro, B., Q. Oppenheim, and J. Zohar, et. al. "Lack of Efficacy of Estrogen Supplementation to Imipramine in Resistant Female Depressives." *Biological Psychiatry*, 1985, 20:576–78.

Sherwin, Barbara B. and Togas Tulandi. "Add-Back: Estrogen Reverses Cognitive Deficits Induced by a Gonadotropin-Releasing Hormone Agonist in Women with Leiomyomata Uteri." *Journal of Clinical Endocrynology and Metabolism*, vol 81, no. 7., July 1996.

Stein, Daniel, et al., Abarbanel Mental Health Center, Bat-Yam, Israel. "Cyclic Psychosis Associated with the Menstrual Cycle." *American Journal of Psychiatry*, March 1993.

Stein, Murray B., M.D., Peter Schmidt, J.M.D., R. David Rubinow, M.D., and Thomas W. Uhde, M.D. "Panic Disorder Patients, Healthy Control Subjects, and Patients With Premenstrual Syndrome." *American Journal of Psychiatry*, 146:10, October 1989.

Studd, John W. W., M.D., and Roger Smith, N.J. "Estrogens and Depression in Women." *Journal of the North American Menopause Society*, vol. 1, no. 1 (1994). Pp. 33–37.

Vliet, Elizabeth Lee, M.D. *Screaming to Be Heard: Hormonal Connections Women Suspect—and Doctors Ignore*. New York: M. Evans, 1995.

Winfrey, Oprah. "Mothers Who Killed Their Children." *The Oprah Winfrey Show*, February 6, 1991.